The Easiest Anti-Inflammatory Diet Cookbook for Beginners:

A **28-Day Meal Plan** Built Around Just **55 Simple & Healthy Ingredients,** Including an Adaptation Week to Reduce Inflammation and Boost Well-Being

MINDFUL MEALS PUBLISHING

2025 Edition

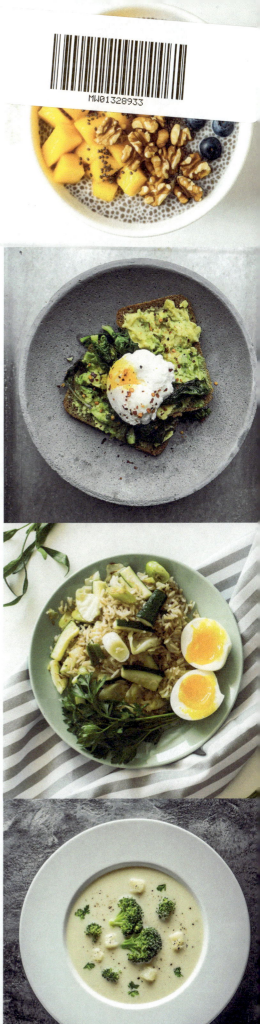

IMPRINT

2nd edition
MINDFUL MEALS PUBLISHING
CONTACT
E-Mail: mindfulmealspublishing@gmail.com

© Copyrights 2025 – All rights reserved

All rights reserved. No part of this book may be copied, distributed, or transmitted in any way without the publisher's prior written consent, with the exception of brief quotations used in critical reviews and certain other noncommercial uses allowed by copyright law. This includes photocopying, recording, and other electronic or mechanical methods.

Legal Notice

This book is intended to provide general information and is designed for educational, personal use only. It is not a replacement for expert counsel. Any negative effects or repercussions arising from the information presented in this book are not the responsibility of the publisher or author. All readers are advised to seek medical advice before making any dietary or lifestyle changes.

Disclaimer Notice

The information contained in this book is for informational purposes only. The publisher and author have done everything possible to guarantee the accuracy and completeness of the information provided. However, they assume no responsibility for errors, inaccuracies, omissions, or any inconsistencies herein. The dietary and lifestyle suggestions outlined in this book may not be suitable for everyone. Individual results may vary, and readers are encouraged to speak with a medical expert before beginning any new diet or health program. The publisher and author both disclaim any liability for any loss or harm, whether caused by direct or indirect means, through the application of any contained information in this book.

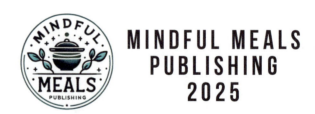

MINDFUL MEALS
PUBLISHING
2025

TABLE OF CONTENTS

INTRODUCTION 6
WHO THIS BOOK IS FOR 6
SOMETHING UNIQUE ABOUT THE BOOK.6

THEORY 8
WHAT IS INFLAMMATION 8
How Inflammation Manifests in the Body 8
What Types of Inflammation Are Dangerous 8
What Factors Trigger Inflammation 8
WAYS TO COMBAT INFLAMMATION 9
FOOD: THE FIRST STEP TO A LIFE WITHOUT INFLAMMATION 9
Which Foods Reduce Inflammation 9
Healthy Cooking Methods 10
Foods to Avoid 10
Common Food Allergens 10
Gentle Transition to an Anti-Inflammatory Diet ..11
55 SIMPLEST ANTI-INFLAMMATORY INGREDIENTS 11
GET YOUR WEEKLY SHOPPING LISTS 11

28-DAY MEAL PLAN 12

BREAKFASTS 15
HEALTHY PORRIDGES AND OATMEAL .16
Quinoa and Blueberry Porridge 16
Oatmeal with Almonds and Berries....................16
Buckwheat Porridge with Pumpkin Seeds and Apples 17
Oatmeal with Spinach and Avocado.................17
EGG DISHES WITH VEGETABLES 18
Spinach and Mushroom Egg Scramble 18
Kale and Tomato Frittata 18
Broccoli and Red Bell Pepper Omelet 19
Sweet Potato and Kale Breakfast Hash 19
SMOOTHIES AND BOWLS 20
Berry Almond Smoothie Bowl 20
Tropical Mango Smoothie 20
Green Avocado Smoothie Bowl 21
Banana and Kale Smoothie 21
PANCAKES AND FRITTERS 22
Buckwheat Pancakes with Blueberries 22
Sweet Potato Fritters 22
Spinach and Chickpea Pancakes 23
Carrot and Zucchini Fritters 23
CRISPY AND DELICIOUS TOASTS 24
Avocado and Tomato Toast 24
Spinach and Egg Toast 24
Chickpea and Avocado Toast 25
Sweet Potato and Avocado Toast 25
LIGHT BREAKFASTS WITH FRUITS AND NUTS 26
Greek Yogurt with Berries and Almonds 26
Chia Pudding with Mango and Walnuts 26
Oatmeal with Bananas and Sunflower Seeds ...27
Quinoa Breakfast Bowl with Apples and Flax Seeds 27

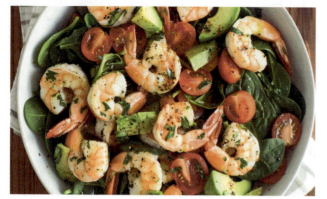

SALADS WITH ANTI-INFLAMMATORY INGREDIENTS 28

SALADS WITH MEAT 29
Chicken and Avocado Salad 29
Turkey and Kale Salad 29
Beef and Broccoli Salad 30
Chicken and Spinach Salad 30
Turkey and Avocado Salad 31
Beef and Sweet Potato Salad 31

SALADS WITH SEAFOOD 32
Salmon and Avocado Salad 32
Shrimp and Quinoa Salad 32
Mackerel and Kale Salad 33
Herring and Beet Salad 33
Salmon and Broccoli Salad 34
Shrimp and Avocado Salad 34

VEGETARIAN & VEGAN SALADS 35
Quinoa and Black Bean Salad 35
Lentil and Roasted Vegetable Salad 35
Chickpea and Avocado Salad 36
Tofu and Kale Salad 36
Tempeh and Wild Rice Salad 37
Cauliflower and Artichoke Salad 37
Lentil and Spinach Salad 38
Chickpea and Kale Salad 38
Black Bean and Avocado Salad 39

Red Bean and Sweet Potato Salad 39
Quinoa and Roasted Vegetable Salad 40
Wild Rice and Kale Salad 40
Barley and Beet Salad 41
Buckwheat and Avocado Salad 41

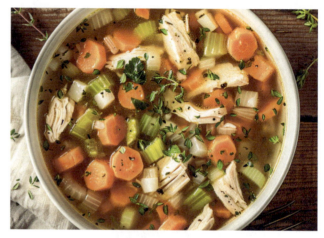

LIGHT SOUPS AND BROTHS 42

MEAT BROTHS AND LIGHT SOUPS 43
Chicken and Vegetable Broth 43
Turkey and Wild Rice Soup 43
Beef and Barley Soup 44
Chicken and Quinoa Soup 44
Turkey and Vegetable Broth 45
Chicken and Cauliflower Soup 45

SEAFOOD SOUPS 46
Salmon and Kale Soup 46
Shrimp and Quinoa Soup 46
Mackerel and Vegetable Soup 47
Herring and Sweet Potato Soup 47
Shrimp and Avocado Soup 48
Salmon and Pumpkin Soup 48

CREAM SOUPS 49
Creamy Broccoli and Spinach Soup 49
Creamy Cauliflower and Garlic Soup 49
Creamy Pumpkin and Carrot Soup 50
Creamy Sweet Potato and Red Pepper Soup 50

Creamy Zucchini and Basil Soup 51

Creamy Tomato and Red Pepper Soup 51

MAIN DISHES 52

FISH AND SEAFOOD DISHES 53
Baked Salmon with Quinoa and Spinach 53

Shrimp and Vegetable Stir-Fry 53

Mackerel with Sweet Potato and Kale 54

Egg-Based Salmon Casserole 54

LEAN MEAT DISHES 55
Grilled Chicken with Quinoa and Avocado 55

Baked Turkey Meatballs with Sweet Potato 55

Chicken and Vegetable Stir-Fry 56

Turkey and Kale Stuffed Peppers 56

Beef and Broccoli Stir-Fry 57

Chicken and Lentil Stew 57

VEGETARIAN DISHES 58
Stuffed Bell Peppers with Black Beans and Corn 58

Chickpea and Sweet Potato Stew 58

Lentil and Vegetable Stew 59

Chickpea and Sweet Potato Curry 59

Black Bean and Sweet Potato Enchiladas (with Tomato Sauce) 60

Quinoa and Vegetable Pilaf 60

Wild Rice and Mushroom Casserole 61

Barley and Spinach Stuffed Peppers 61

BAKING AND DESSERTS 62

GLUTEN-FREE BAKING 63
Almond Flour Blueberry Muffins 63

Buckwheat Banana Bread 63

Pumpkin and Oat Cookies 64

Buckwheat and Carrot Cake 64

BAKING WITH WHOLE GRAIN FLOUR ...65
Whole Grain Flour Banana Muffins 65

Whole Grain Carrot Cake 65

Whole Grain Pumpkin Bread 66

Whole Grain Apple Cinnamon Muffins 66

NUT AND SEED DESSERTS 67
Almond Flour Chocolate Chip Cookies 67

Chia Seed Pudding with Berries 67

Walnut and Date Energy Balls 68

Flaxseed and Blueberry Muffins 68

PLANT-BASED MILK DESSERTS 69
Almond Milk Quinoa Pudding 69

Coconut Milk Chia Pudding 69

Oat Milk Chocolate Pudding 70

Almond Milk Berry Popsicles 70

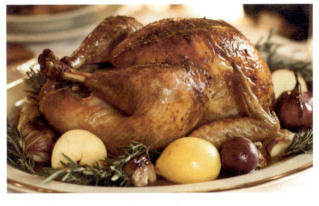

FESTIVE DISHES TAILORED FOR AN ANTI-INFLAMMATORY DIET 71

A NOTE OF THANKS 82

INTRODUCTION

WHO THIS BOOK IS FOR

This book is designed for anyone looking to take control of their health by reducing inflammation through diet. Whether you're new to an anti-inflammatory diet or have some experience but need a structured approach, this book will guide you through the process.

If you're struggling with chronic conditions like arthritis, heart disease, or autoimmune disorders, this book offers a ray of hope. The meal plans and recipes are written with the intention of helping to alleviate symptoms, empowering you to manage inflammation and improve your health through nutrition.

This book is a valuable resource even if you don't have a specific health condition but are interested in preventing chronic diseases and maintaining optimal health. The anti-inflammatory diet is not just for those who are already sick; it's a proactive approach to health that can benefit anyone.

Moreover, this book is an ideal companion for those with a busy lifestyle who aspire to eat healthily but have limited time for meal preparation. The recipes are straightforward, require minimal ingredients, and are designed to be quick and easy to prepare, facilitating adherence to a healthy eating plan.

This book is a friendly companion for anyone who is interested in living a life that is both healthier and more vibrant by embracing an anti-inflammatory diet. No matter your starting point, this book is here to support and guide you every step of the way.

SOMETHING UNIQUE ABOUT THE BOOK

Unique and Delicious Recipes!
Our book offers a wide selection of recipes to satisfy any taste – whether you're in the mood for a light, refreshing breakfast or a savory main dish, a meat lover or a vegetarian!

What's more, we've made sure to include a mouthwatering range of gluten-free and whole-grain dessert options. No matter what your dietary preferences are, our book is designed to provide a comprehensive meal plan, giving you the freedom to explore and experiment. We're confident you'll discover some new culinary favorites that cater to your unique tastes.

Only the Healthiest and Most Accessible Ingredients!
Our goal in creating this book was to make it practical and accessible for everyday use. No more overwhelming meal plans with endless ingredients! No more recipes with items that are impossible to find in your local store!

We've thoughtfully designed a nutrition plan that focuses on the most essential, nutritious, readily available ingredients, ensuring that healthy eating is simple and satisfying.

28-Day Meal Plan with an Adaptation Week.

You'll find a carefully crafted 28-day meal plan that follows the principles of an anti-inflammatory diet, designed to support your health and provide balanced nutrition.

The book includes a special adaptation week to help you transition smoothly and stress-free into this new way of eating, giving you time to adjust gradually.

In addition, a shopping list is included for each week of the meal plan. It is available in two formats: a printable version for traditional use and a mobile app-ready version, making it easy to plan your groceries on the go.

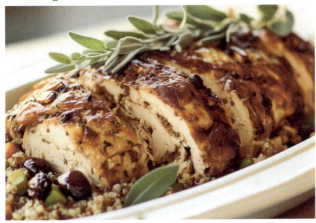

Special Edition: The Holiday Recipes!

In this special section of the book, you'll find 10 delightful holiday recipes designed to bring flavor and health to your Thanksgiving table. Whether you're looking to prepare the perfect roast turkey with a healthier twist or a flavorful tofu turkey alternative, these recipes are crafted with anti-inflammatory ingredients to ensure that your holiday meal supports your well-being.

From savory main courses to indulgent yet nutritious holiday pies, this chapter has everything you need to impress your guests.

Each recipe uses whole foods and spices like turmeric and ginger to maximize flavor while minimizing inflammation. Get ready to enjoy the holidays with these easy-to-follow, delicious dishes that make no compromise on taste or health.

Perfect for anyone who enjoys traditional holiday meals while mindful of their dietary choices!

Colorful Images for Every Dish!

What's a cookbook without vibrant photos of the delicious dishes? Our images are designed to inspire your culinary creativity and give you a clear idea of what the finished dish should look like. Every recipe is paired with a bright, delicious image to make following the instructions easier and help you achieve the perfect result. The visual aspect is a crucial part of the cooking and dining experience, and we've made sure that each photo captures the whole appeal and variety of our recipes, helping you create culinary masterpieces in your kitchen.

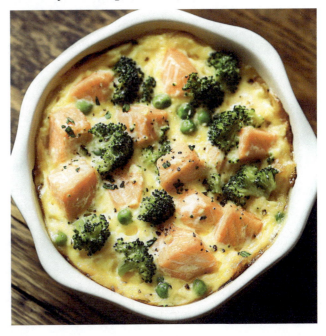

THEORY

WHAT IS INFLAMMATION

How Inflammation Manifests in the Body.

The normal response of the body to an injury or infection is inflammation, which serves as a defensive mechanism to heal and repair damaged tissues. When something harmful or irritating affects a part of your body, the immune system releases white blood cells and substances known as cytokines to protect the area. This process often results in visible signs such as redness, swelling, heat, and pain. Acute inflammation is usually short-term, lasting only a few days, and is crucial for healing. For example, when you sprain your ankle, the area swells and becomes red when your body is working to heal the tissue that has been destroyed. If the process works correctly, the inflammation subsides once the threat is neutralized and healing begins. However, in chronic inflammation, these cellular processes become dysregulated, leading to ongoing tissue damage and the potential for disease.

What Types of Inflammation Are Dangerous.

Although acute inflammation is an essential component of the healing process, chronic inflammation is where the danger lies.
Unlike acute inflammation, chronic inflammation can occur without a clear cause, sometimes due to the immune system mistakenly attacking health issues. Chronic inflammation, a silent but significant contributor to many health issues, can lead to a range of serious diseases. In autoimmune conditions like rheumatoid arthritis, the autoimmune response targets the joints, resulting in discomfort and inflammation and eventually leading to joint destruction. In cardiovascular disorders, persistent inflammation is crucial in the pathogenesis of atherosclerosis, where the walls of arteries become thickened with plaque, increasing the risk of heart attacks and strokes. Chronic inflammation is also linked to the development of certain cancers, as the constant state of inflammation can cause DNA damage and promote the proliferation of abnormal cells. Moreover, low-grade chronic inflammation, which may not present any immediate symptoms, is involved in the pathogenesis of insulin resistance, type 2 diabetes, and obesity. This type of inflammation can silently damage various organs and tissues over time, highlighting the importance of addressing inflammation before it leads to more severe health problems.

What Factors Trigger Inflammation.

Several factors can trigger inflammation, from infections and injuries to lifestyle choices and environmental exposures. One of the most common triggers is bacteria, viruses, or fungi infection. For example, bacterial infections can lead to the release of toxins that cause tissue damage, prompting an inflammatory response. Injuries, such as cuts, burns, or fractures, also trigger inflammation as the body works to repair damaged tissues. Beyond these apparent causes, lifestyle factors play a significant role in promoting chronic inflammation. Poor diet, characterized by high sugar, refined carbohydrates, and trans fats, can lead to metabolic disturbances and promote low-grade inflammation. Lack of physical activity is another contributor, as exercise on a regular basis helps you stay healthy and reduce inflammation. Chronic stress and poor sleep can also trigger or exacerbate inflammation by disrupting the balance of stress hormones and immune function. Elements of the environment can further contribute to an inflammatory state, including but not limited to exposure to pollution, chemicals, and allergens. Comprehension of these triggers is essential for the management and prevention of inflammation, emphasizing the need for a comprehensive strategy for health that incorporates exercise, nutrition, stress reduction, and reducing exposure to harmful substances.

WAYS TO COMBAT INFLAMMATION

Reducing inflammation in the body requires a multifaceted strategy that incorporates dietary modifications, lifestyle tweaks, and stress management. One of the most effective strategies is adopting an anti-inflammatory diet that is abundant in fruits, vegetables, lean meats, and healthy fats, including omega-3 fatty acids found in fish and flaxseeds. These foods help reduce inflammation by supplying essential nutrients and antioxidants that fight oxidative stress. Sport promotes better circulation, helping to clear out inflammatory substances from the bloodstream. Stress management is equally essential since chronic stress can exacerbate inflammation. Practices including yoga, deep breathing techniques, and meditation can help alleviate tension and reduce inflammation. Furthermore, good quality sleep is absolutely essential since poor sleep can increase the body's inflammatory response. Including these techniques in your everyday schedule will effectively combat inflammation and improve your overall health.

FOOD: THE FIRST STEP TO A LIFE WITHOUT INFLAMMATION

Which Foods Reduce Inflammation.
The foundation of an anti-inflammatory diet is built upon foods that are scientifically proven to naturally reduce inflammation in the body. These consist of an extensive array of fruits and vegetables abundant in antioxidants and phytonutrients. Berries, such as blueberries, strawberries, and raspberries, are packed with anthocyanins, which have strong anti-inflammatory effects. Leafy greens like spinach, kale, and Swiss chard are high in vitamins A, C, and K, all of which support the immune system and help fight inflammation. Omega-3 fatty acids, found in considerable quantities within the category of fatty fish (including

salmon, mackerel, and sardines), walnuts, and flaxseeds, are considered healthy lipids and are crucial as they directly reduce the production of inflammatory molecules. Nutrient-dense grains like quinoa, brown rice, and oats, as well as nuts, seeds, and legumes, deliver dietary fiber, a vital component for maintaining optimal gut health and mitigating inflammation inside the digestive system. By regularly incorporating these scientifically-backed foods into your diet, you can significantly lower your body's inflammatory response.

Healthy Cooking Methods.
Even the healthiest foods can lose their anti-inflammatory benefits if not adequately prepared. To enhance your diet's anti-inflammatory benefits, choose cooking methods that retain nutrients and minimize the creation of harmful substances. Steaming, sautéing, and roasting at moderate temperatures are excellent ways to cook vegetables while retaining their vitamins and minerals. Grilling and broiling can be healthy if done at lower temperatures to prevent charring, which can create inflammatory compounds called advanced glycation end-products (AGEs). Slow-cooking methods, such as braising and simmering, are also beneficial, particularly for preparing meats and legumes, as they help to preserve their nutrient content while reducing the risk of creating harmful compounds. Healthy cooking oils, like olive oil and avocado oil, which are high in monounsaturated fats, also support the anti-inflammatory process. By choosing these cooking methods, you enhance the nutritional value of your meals and ensure that your diet is genuinely anti-inflammatory.

Foods to Avoid.
To effectively combat inflammation, it's just as important to know which foods to avoid as it is to know which to include. Highly processed foods are among the biggest culprits in triggering inflammation. These include foods high in refined sugars, such as sugary snacks, sodas, and candies, and refined carbohydrates, like white bread and pastries. Trans fatty acids, present in numerous fried and commercially baked products, are particularly harmful as they increase inflammation and contribute to heart disease. Red meat, especially when processed, can also promote inflammation, mainly when consumed in large quantities. Specific culinary techniques, such as deep frying, can also create harmful compounds that trigger inflammation. Reducing or eliminating these foods can significantly lower inflammation levels and improve overall health.

Common Food Allergens.
Food allergies and sensitivities can be hidden contributors to chronic inflammation, as they cause the immune system to react negatively to specific proteins in foods. Common allergens include gluten, found in wheat, barley, rye, and dairy products, particularly in patients with lactose intolerance or a sensitivity to casein. Other common allergens include soy, eggs, peanuts, tree nuts, and shellfish. Even if you do not have a diagnosed allergy,

mild sensitivities to these foods can still cause inflammation, leading to symptoms like bloating, headaches, or joint pain. If you suspect food sensitivity, it can be helpful to try an elimination diet under the guidance of a healthcare professional. Minimizing possible allergens from your diet and systematically reintroducing them can help identify any inflammation-related triggers.

Gentle Transition to an Anti-Inflammatory Diet.
Adopting an anti-inflammatory diet doesn't have to be overwhelming. Making small, gradual changes can help your body adjust without feeling deprived. Begin by including a greater variety of anti-inflammatory foods in your meals, such as adding a handful of berries to your breakfast or a leafy green salad with your dinner. Step by step, decrease your consumption of processed foods and replace them with whole, nutrient-dense alternatives. If you're used to eating much red meat, try introducing more plant-based proteins like beans, lentils, or tofu.
Additionally, experiment with new cooking methods that preserve the nutritional content of your food, such as steaming or roasting. Slowly taking these steps allows your palate and body to adapt, making it easier to maintain these long-term changes. Over time, these small shifts will lead to a more balanced diet that naturally reduces inflammation and supports better health.

55 SIMPLEST ANTI-INFLAMMATORY INGREDIENTS

We have carefully selected **55 of the most popular and essential anti-inflammatory ingredients** to serve as the foundation of our meal plan. Each ingredient was chosen not only for its well-known health benefits but also for its accessibility and versatility in everyday cooking. In addition to these core 55 ingredients, we have also included anti-inflammatory spices and herbs. By incorporating these powerful ingredients, we've created a balanced and easy-to-follow plan that supports your journey toward reducing inflammation and improving overall well-being.

GET YOUR WEEKLY SHOPPING LISTS

For your convenience, we've prepared a bonus shopping list in two different formats: a PDF for printing, and a Google Sheet for copying to your mobile app!

Scan the barcode to access the printable PDF file and Google Sheet.

28-DAY MEAL PLAN WITH AN ADAPTATION WEEK

The **adaptation week is the first step in transitioning to an anti-inflammatory diet**, designed to gently ease your body into new dietary habits. This week serves as a buffer, allowing your body to adjust without overwhelming changes, reducing the chances of stress or discomfort as you move toward healthier eating.

During this week, here's what you'll focus on:

1. **Gradual Reduction of Inflammatory Foods**: You'll slowly reduce industrialized foods, processed sugars, and trans fats while adding more anti-inflammatory options like leafy greens, berries, and omega-3-rich fish.
2. **Portion Control**: Instead of cutting out all inflammatory foods at once, reduce portion sizes of foods like red meat or processed snacks while increasing alternatives abundant in dietary fiber, such as whole grains and vegetables.
3. **Boosting Antioxidant Intake**: Start incorporating antioxidant-rich foods like nuts, olive oil, and green tea into your meals. These will help reduce inflammation and support your overall well-being.
4. **Stay Hydrated**: Proper hydration is key. In addition to water, herbal teas like ginger or turmeric can be added to help with the detoxification process and further reduce inflammation.
5. **Exercise and Rest**: Light physical activity, such as walking or yoga, along with good rest, will help support your body's transition, making it easier to adapt to your new eating habits.

Below is a meal plan for the first **adaptation week** of transitioning to an anti-inflammatory diet. It's best to start with breakfasts and gradually add other meals after a few days.

ADAPTATION WEEK

	Breakfast	*Lunch*	*Dinner*
DAY 1	Oatmeal with Almonds and Berries (300 cals) - p.16	Your usual meals	Your usual meals
DAY 2	Broccoli and Red Bell Pepper Omelet (220 cals) - p.19	Your usual meals	Your usual meals
DAY 3	Berry Almond Smoothie Bowl (350 cals) - p.20	Your usual meals	Your usual meals
DAY 4	Spinach and Chickpea Pancakes (240 cals) - p.23	Chicken and Vegetable Broth (250 cals) - p.43	Your usual meals
DAY 5	Spinach and Egg Toast (350 cals) - p.24	Salmon and Kale Soup (250 cals) - p.46	Your usual meals
DAY 6	Chia Pudding with Mango and Walnuts (300 cals) - p.26	Creamy Sweet Potato and Red Pepper Soup (190 cals) - p.50	Turkey and Kale Salad (320 cals) - p.29
DAY 7	Buckwheat Porridge with Pumpkin Seeds and Apples (320 cals) - p.17	Creamy Broccoli and Spinach Soup (150 cals) - p.49	Chicken and Avocado Salad (350 cals) - p.29

28-DAY MEAL PLAN

After the adaptation week, you can begin following the full meal plan. Below, you will find a **28-day meal plan** for each week.

WEEK 1

	Breakfast	Lunch	Dinner
DAY 1	Quinoa and Blueberry Porridge (350 cals) - p.16	Turkey and Wild Rice Soup (300 cals) - p.43 Quinoa and Black Bean Salad (350 cals) - p.35	Baked Salmon with Quinoa and Spinach (450 cals) - p.53
DAY 2	Spinach and Mushroom Egg Scramble (200 cals) - p.18	Shrimp and Quinoa Soup (300 cals) - p.46 Lentil and Roasted Vegetable Salad (400 cals) - p.35	Grilled Chicken with Quinoa and Avocado (450 cals) - p.55
DAY 3	Tropical Mango Smoothie (400 cals) - p.20	Creamy Cauliflower and Garlic Soup (170 cals) - p.49 Salmon and Avocado Salad (400 cals) - p.32	Stuffed Bell Peppers with Black Beans and Corn (350 cals) - p.58
DAY 4	Buckwheat Pancakes with Blueberries (280 cals) - p.22	Beef and Barley Soup (350 cals) - p.44 Chickpea and Avocado Salad (380 cals) - p.36	Chickpea and Sweet Potato Stew (400 cals) - p.58
DAY 5	Avocado and Tomato Toast (300 cals) - p.24	Mackerel and Vegetable Soup (270 cals) - p.47 Tofu and Kale Salad (350 cals) - p.36	Baked Turkey Meatballs with Sweet Potato (400 cals) - p.55
DAY 6	Greek Yogurt with Berries and Almonds (350 cals) - p.26	Creamy Pumpkin and Carrot Soup (180 cals) - p.50 Beef and Broccoli Salad (400 cals) - p.30	Lentil and Vegetable Stew (300 cals) - p.59
DAY 7	Kale and Tomato Frittata (250 cals) - p.18	Chicken and Quinoa Soup (300 cals) - p.44 Tempeh and Wild Rice Salad (400 cals) - p.37	Shrimp and Vegetable Stir-Fry (300 cals) - p.53

WEEK 2

	Breakfast	Lunch	Dinner
DAY 8	Oatmeal with Spinach and Avocado (320 cals) - p.17	Herring and Sweet Potato Soup (280 cals) - p.47 Cauliflower and Artichoke Salad (220 cals) - p.37	Chicken and Vegetable Stir-Fry (350 cals) - p.56
DAY 9	Sweet Potato Fritters (220 cals) - p.22	Creamy Sweet Potato and Red Pepper Soup (190 cals) - p.50 Chicken and Spinach Salad (350 cals) - p.30	Chickpea and Sweet Potato Curry (400 cals) - p.59
DAY 10	Chickpea and Avocado Toast (320 cals) - p.25	Turkey and Vegetable Broth (250 cals) - p.45 Lentil and Spinach Salad (300 cals) - p.38	Black Bean and Sweet Potato Enchiladas (with Tomato Sauce) (400 cals) - p.60
DAY 11	Oatmeal with Bananas and Sunflower Seeds (350 cals) - p.27	Shrimp and Avocado Soup (320 cals) - p.48 Chickpea and Kale Salad (350 cals) - p.38	Turkey and Kale Stuffed Peppers (400 cals) - p.56
DAY 12	Sweet Potato and Kale Breakfast Hash (280 cals) - p.19	Creamy Zucchini and Basil Soup (140 cals) - p.51 Shrimp and Quinoa Salad (350 cals) - p.32	Beef and Broccoli Stir-Fry (350 cals) - p.57
DAY 13	Oatmeal with Almonds and Berries (300 cals) - p.16	Chicken and Cauliflower Soup (240 cals) - p.45 Black Bean and Avocado Salad (380 cals) - p.39	Quinoa and Vegetable Pilaf (350 cals) - p.61
DAY 14	Broccoli and Red Bell Pepper Omelet (220 cals) - p.19	Salmon and Pumpkin Soup (300 cals) - p.48 Red Bean and Sweet Potato Salad (400 cals) - p.39	Wild Rice and Mushroom Casserole (300 cals) - p.61

WEEK 3

	Breakfast	Lunch	Dinner
DAY 15	Buckwheat Porridge with Pumpkin Seeds and Apples (320 cals) - p.17	Creamy Tomato and Red Pepper Soup (160 cals) - p.51 Turkey and Avocado Salad (350 cals) - p.31	Mackerel with Sweet Potato and Kale (400 cals) - p.54
DAY 16	Banana and Kale Smoothie (350 cals) - p.21	Chicken and Vegetable Broth (250 cals) - p.43 Mackerel and Kale Salad (370 cals) - p.33	Barley and Spinach Stuffed Peppers (300 cals) - p.60
DAY 17	Carrot and Zucchini Fritters (240 cals) - p.23	Salmon and Kale Soup (250 cals) - p.46 Quinoa and Roasted Vegetable Salad (350 cals) - p.40	Chicken and Lentil Stew (400 cals) - p.57
DAY 18	Sweet Potato and Avocado Toast (340 cals) - p.25	Creamy Broccoli and Spinach Soup (150 cals) - p.49 Herring and Beet Salad (380 cals) - p.33	Egg-Based Salmon Casserole (280 cals) - p.54
DAY 19	Quinoa Breakfast Bowl with Apples and Flax Seeds (400 cals) - p.27	Turkey and Wild Rice Soup (300 cals) - p.43 Wild Rice and Kale Salad (400 cals) - p.40	Stuffed Bell Peppers with Black Beans and Corn (350 cals) - p.58
DAY 20	Spinach and Mushroom Egg Scramble (200 cals) - p.18	Shrimp and Quinoa Soup (300 cals) - p.46 Barley and Beet Salad (420 cals) - p.41	Chickpea and Sweet Potato Stew (400 cals) - p.58
DAY 21	Quinoa and Blueberry Porridge (350 cals) - p.16	Creamy Cauliflower and Garlic Soup (170 cals) - p.49 Beef and Sweet Potato Salad (400 cals) - p.31	Shrimp and Vegetable Stir-Fry (300 cals) - p.53

WEEK 4

	Breakfast	Lunch	Dinner
DAY 22	Kale and Tomato Frittata (250 cals) - p.18	Beef and Barley Soup (350 cals) - p.44 Buckwheat and Avocado Salad (360 cals) - p.41	Lentil and Vegetable Stew (300 cals) - p.59
DAY 23	Berry Almond Smoothie Bowl (350 cals) - p.20	Mackerel and Vegetable Soup (270 cals) - p.47 Chicken and Avocado Salad (350 cals) - p.29	Chickpea and Sweet Potato Curry (400 cals) - p.59
DAY 24	Spinach and Chickpea Pancakes (240 cals) - p.23	Creamy Pumpkin and Carrot Soup (180 cals) - p.50 Salmon and Broccoli Salad (400 cals) - p.34	Grilled Chicken with Quinoa and Avocado (450 cals) - p.55
DAY 25	Oatmeal with Spinach and Avocado (320 cals) - p.17	Chicken and Quinoa Soup (300 cals) - p.44 Shrimp and Avocado Salad (380 cals) - p.34	Black Bean and Sweet Potato Enchiladas (with Tomato Sauce) (400 cals) - p.60
DAY 26	Spinach and Egg Toast (350 cals) - p.24	Shrimp and Avocado Soup (320 cals) - p.48 Tofu and Kale Salad (350 cals) - p.36	Baked Turkey Meatballs with Sweet Potato (400 cals) - p.55
DAY 27	Chia Pudding with Mango and Walnuts (300 cals) - p.26	Creamy Zucchini and Basil Soup (140 cals) - p.51 Turkey and Kale Salad (320 cals) - p.29	Baked Salmon with Quinoa and Spinach (450 cals) - p.53
DAY 28	Sweet Potato and Kale Breakfast Hash (280 cals) - p.19	Turkey and Vegetable Broth (250 cals) - p.45 Chickpea and Kale Salad (350 cals) - p.38	Quinoa and Vegetable Pilaf (350 cals) - p.61

Please note that since everyone is different and requires an individual caloric intake, our meal plan offers a foundational solution. Be sure to consult a specialist to determine your specific calorie needs, and adjust your meals by adding extra snacks as necessary.

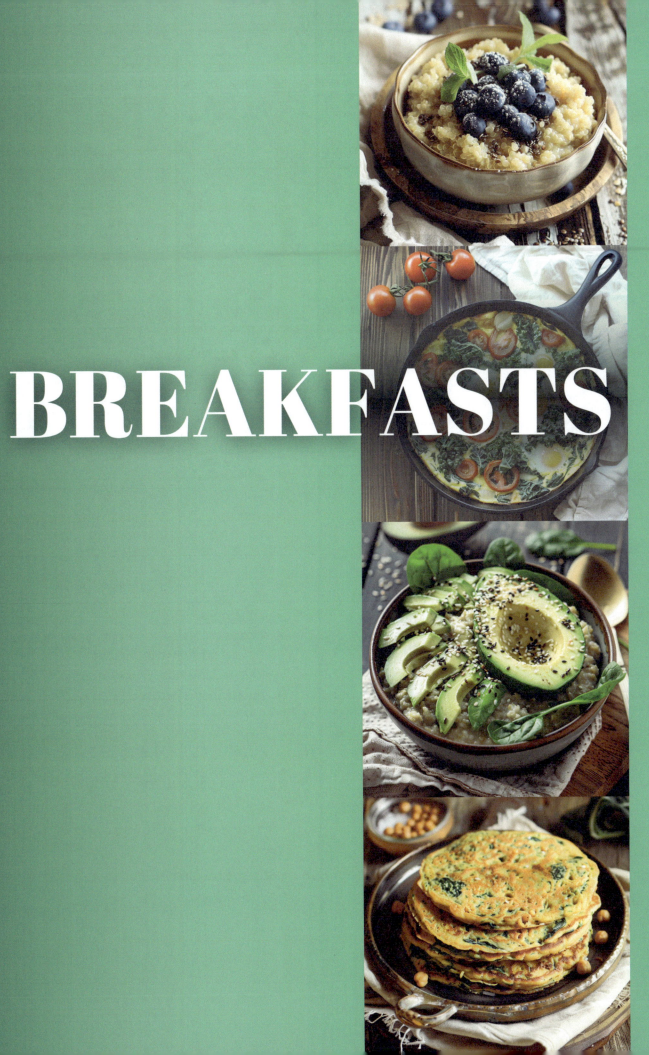

BREAKFASTS

Healthy Porridges and Oatmeal

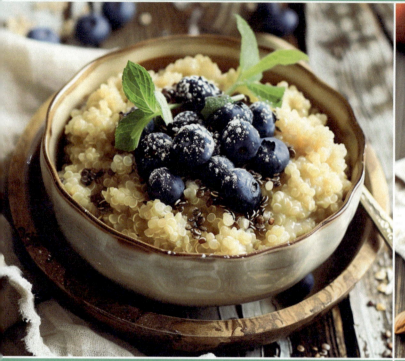

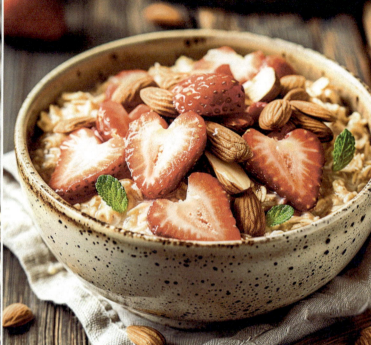

Quinoa and Blueberry Porridge

2 | 20 min | Macronutrients (per serving): Calories: 350 | Protein: 12 g Fat: 10 g Carbs: 55 g

INGREDIENTS

- 1 cup quinoa
- 2 cups almond milk
- 1 cup blueberries
- 1 tablespoon chia seeds
- 1 tablespoon flax seeds

Allergens:
- Nuts (almond milk)

DIRECTIONS

1. Rinse the quinoa under cold water.
2. In a medium saucepan, combine quinoa and almond milk. Bring to a boil.
3. Reduce heat and simmer for about 15 minutes, or until quinoa is tender and liquid is absorbed.
4. Stir in blueberries, chia seeds, and flax seeds.
5. Serve warm.

Oatmeal with Almonds and Berries

2 | 10 min | Macronutrients (per serving): Calories: 300 | Protein: 8 g Fat: 12 g Carbs: 45 g

INGREDIENTS

- 1 cup oats
- 2 cups water
- 1/2 cup strawberries, sliced
- 1/4 cup almonds, chopped
- 1 tablespoon flax seeds

Allergens:
- Nuts (almonds)

DIRECTIONS

1. In a medium saucepan, bring water to a boil.
2. Add oats and reduce heat to a simmer. Cook for about 5-7 minutes, or until the oats are tender.
3. Stir in strawberries, almonds, and flax seeds.
4. Serve warm.

Healthy Porridges and Oatmeal

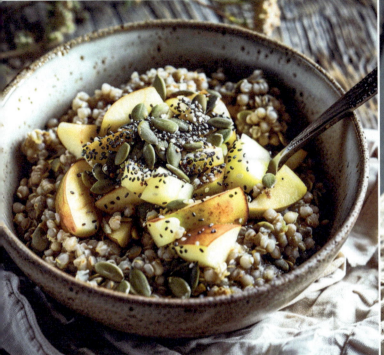

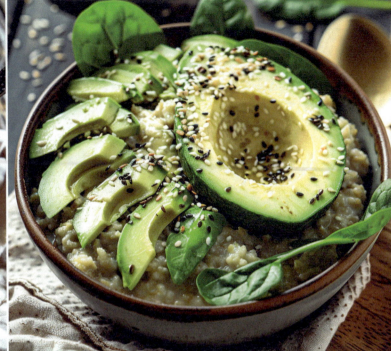

Buckwheat Porridge with Pumpkin Seeds and Apples

Serves: 2 | Time: 20 min

Macronutrients (per serving):
Calories: 320 | Protein: 10 g | Fat: 10 g | Carbs: 50 g

INGREDIENTS

- 1 cup buckwheat groats
- 2 cups water
- 1 apple, diced
- 1/4 cup pumpkin seeds
- 1 tablespoon chia seeds

Allergens:
- None

DIRECTIONS

1. Rinse buckwheat groats under cold water.
2. In a medium saucepan, combine buckwheat and water. Bring to a boil.
3. Reduce heat and simmer for about 15 minutes, or until buckwheat is tender.
4. Stir in diced apple, pumpkin seeds, and chia seeds.
5. Serve warm.

Oatmeal with Spinach and Avocado

Serves: 2 | Time: 10 min

Macronutrients (per serving):
Calories: 320 | Protein: 8 g | Fat: 16 g | Carbs: 40 g

INGREDIENTS

- 1 cup oats
- 2 cups water
- 1 cup spinach, chopped
- 1 avocado, sliced
- 1 tablespoon flax seeds

Allergens:
- None

DIRECTIONS

1. In a medium saucepan, bring water to a boil.
2. Add oats and reduce heat to a simmer. Cook for about 5-7 minutes, or until the oats are tender.
3. Stir in chopped spinach and cook for another 2 minutes.
4. Top with sliced avocado and flax seeds.
5. Serve warm.

Egg Dishes with Vegetables

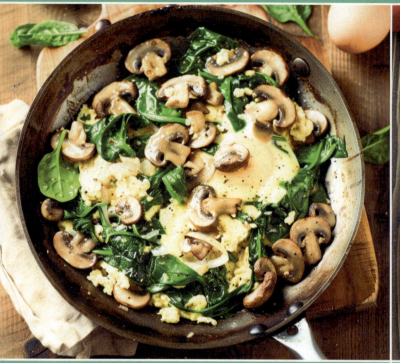

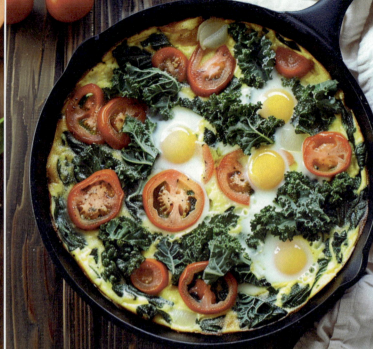

Spinach and Mushroom Egg Scramble

| 2 | 15 min | Macronutrients (per serving): Calories: 200 | Protein: 14 g Fat: 14 g Carbs: 6 g |

INGREDIENTS

- 3 eggs
- 1 cup spinach, chopped
- 1/2 cup mushrooms, sliced
- 1/4 cup onions, diced
- 1 tablespoon olive oil (optional for cooking)

Allergens:
- Eggs

DIRECTIONS

1. Heat olive oil in a skillet over medium heat.
2. Add onions and cook until translucent, about 3 min.
3. Add mushrooms and cook for another 5 minutes until softened.
4. Add spinach and cook until wilted, about 2 minutes.
5. Beat the eggs in a bowl and pour them into the skillet.
6. Stir continuously until the eggs are fully cooked.
7. Serve warm.

Kale and Tomato Frittata

| 2 | 25 min | Macronutrients (per serving): Calories: 250 | Protein: 16 g Fat: 18 g Carbs: 8 g |

INGREDIENTS

- 4 eggs
- 1 cup kale, chopped
- 1/2 cup tomatoes, diced
- 1/4 cup onions, diced
- 1 tablespoon olive oil (optional for cooking)

Allergens:
- Eggs

DIRECTIONS

1. Preheat the oven to 375°F (190°C).
2. Heat olive oil in an oven-safe skillet over medium heat.
3. Add onions and cook until translucent, about 3 min.
4. Add kale and cook until wilted, about 3 minutes
5. . Add tomatoes and cook for 2 more minutes.
6. Beat eggs in a bowl and pour over the vegetables.
7. Transfer the skillet to the oven and bake for 10-12 minutes, or until eggs are set. Serve warm.

Egg Dishes with Vegetables

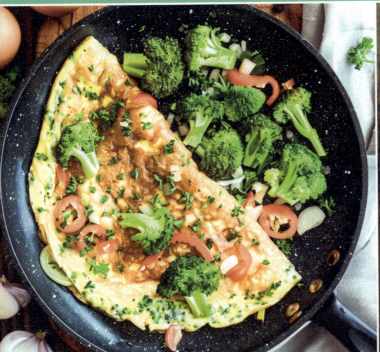
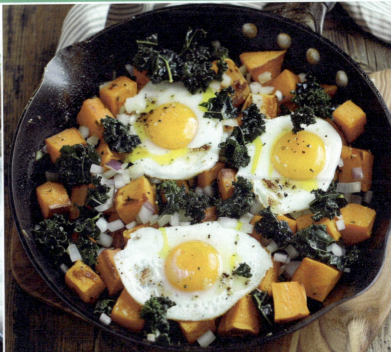

Broccoli and Red Bell Pepper Omelet

🍴 2 ⏲ 15 min Macronutrients (per serving): Calories: 220 Protein: 14 g Fat: 16 g Carbs: 6 g

INGREDIENTS

- 3 eggs
- 1/4 cup onions, diced
- 1/2 red bell pepper, diced
- 1/2 cup broccoli florets, chopped
- 1 tablespoon olive oil (optional for cooking)

Allergens:
- Eggs

DIRECTIONS

1. Heat olive oil in a skillet over medium heat.
2. Add onions and cook until translucent, about 3 min.
3. Add broccoli and red bell pepper and cook for another 5 minutes until tender.
4. Beat the eggs in a bowl and pour them into the skillet.
5. Cook until the eggs start to set, then fold the omelet in half.
6. Continue cooking until the eggs are fully cooked.
7. Serve warm.

Sweet Potato and Kale Breakfast Hash

🍴 2 ⏲ 20 min Macronutrients (per serving): Calories: 280 Protein: 10 g Fat: 12 g Carbs: 32 g

INGREDIENTS

- 2 eggs
- 1 sweet potato, peeled and diced
- 1 cup kale, chopped
- 1/4 cup onions, diced
- 1 tablespoon olive oil (optional for cooking)

Allergens:
- Eggs

DIRECTIONS

1. Heat olive oil in a skillet over medium heat.
2. Add onions and cook until translucent, about 3 minutes.
3. Add sweet potatoes and cook until tender, about 10 minutes.
4. Add kale and cook until wilted, about 3 minutes.
5. In a separate skillet, cook the eggs to your preference (scrambled, fried, etc.).
6. Serve the eggs over the sweet potato and kale hash.

Smoothies and Bowls

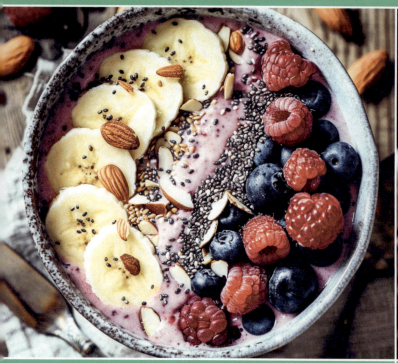

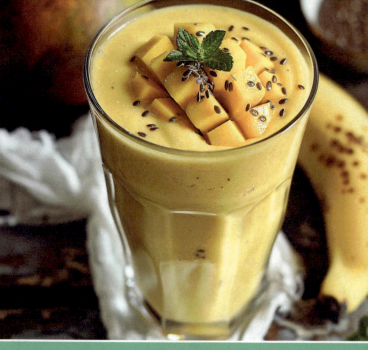

Berry Almond Smoothie Bowl

		Macronutrients (per serving):	Protein: 8 g
1	5 min	Calories: 350	Fat: 18 g Carbs: 45 g

INGREDIENTS

- 1 cup mixed berries
- 1 banana
- 1/2 cup almond milk
- 2 tablespoons chia seeds
- 1/4 cup almonds, chopped

Allergens:
- Nuts (almonds)

DIRECTIONS

1. In a blender, combine mixed berries, banana, and almond milk. Blend until smooth.
2. Pour the smoothie into a bowl.
3. Top with chia seeds and chopped almonds.
4. Serve immediately.

Tropical Mango Smoothie

		Macronutrients (per serving):	Protein: 10 g
1	5 min	Calories: 400	Fat: 20 g Carbs: 50 g

INGREDIENTS

- 1 mango, peeled and diced
- 1 banana
- 1 cup coconut milk
- 2 tablespoons flax seeds
- 1/4 cup Greek yogurt

Allergens:
- Dairy (Greek yogurt)

DIRECTIONS

1. In a blender, combine mango, banana, coconut milk, and Greek yogurt. Blend until smooth.
2. Pour the smoothie into a glass.
3. Stir in flax seeds.
4. Serve immediately

Smoothies and Bowls

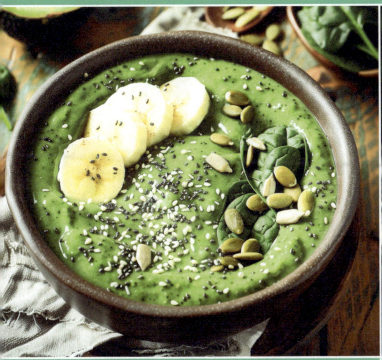

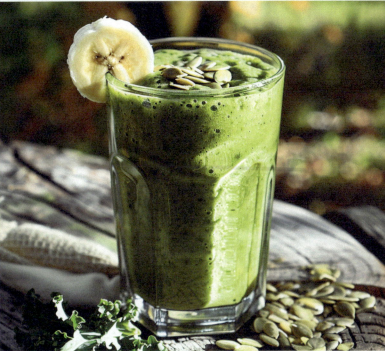

Green Avocado Smoothie Bowl

| 🍴 1 | 🕐 5 min | Macronutrients (per serving): Calories: 380 | Protein: 8 g Fat: 28 g Carbs: 30 g |

INGREDIENTS

- 1 avocado
- 1 cup spinach
- 1 banana
- 1 cup almond milk
- 2 tablespoons sunflower seeds

Allergens:
- Nuts (almond milk)
- Seeds (sunflower seeds)

DIRECTIONS

1. In a blender, combine avocado, spinach, banana, and almond milk. Blend until smooth.
2. Pour the smoothie into a bowl.
3. Top with sunflower seeds.
4. Serve immediately.

Banana and Kale Smoothie

| 🍴 1 | 🕐 5 min | Macronutrients (per serving): Calories: 350 | Protein: 12 g Fat: 15 g Carbs: 40 g |

INGREDIENTS

- 1 banana
- 1 cup kale, chopped
- 1 cup oat milk
- 2 tablespoons pumpkin seeds
- 1/4 cup Greek yogurt

Allergens:
- Dairy (Greek yogurt)

DIRECTIONS

1. In a blender, combine banana, kale, oat milk, and Greek yogurt. Blend until smooth.
2. Pour the smoothie into a glass.
3. Stir in pumpkin seeds.
4. Serve immediately.

Pancakes and Fritters

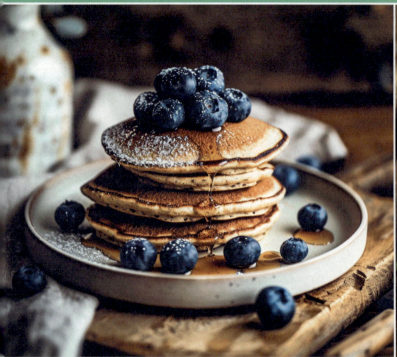
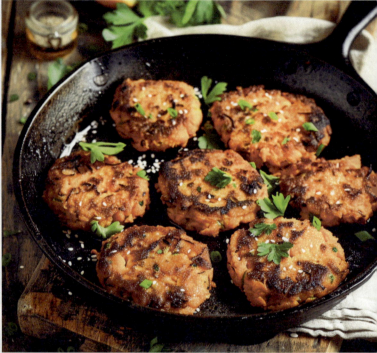

Buckwheat Pancakes with Blueberries

| 2 | 15 min | Macronutrients (per serving): Calories: 280 | Protein: 9 g Fat: 8 g Carbs: 45 g |

INGREDIENTS

- 1 cup buckwheat flour
- 1 cup almond milk
- 1 egg
- 1 cup blueberries
- 2 tablespoons chia seeds

Allergens:
- Nuts (almond milk)
- Eggs

DIRECTIONS

1. In a mixing bowl, combine buckwheat flour, almond milk, and egg. Mix until smooth.
2. Gently fold in the blueberries and chia seeds.
3. Heat a non-stick skillet over medium heat. Pour 1/4 cup of batter onto the skillet for each pancake.
4. Cook until bubbles form on the surface, then flip and cook until golden brown, about 2-3 minutes per side.
5. Serve warm.

Sweet Potato Fritters

| 2 | 20 min | Macronutrients (per serving): Calories: 220 | Protein: 10 g Fat: 8 g Carbs: 35 g |

INGREDIENTS

- 1 large sweet potato, grated
- 2 eggs
- 1/4 cup onions, finely diced
- 2 tablespoons flax seeds
- 1/4 cup whole grain flour

Allergens:
- Eggs
- Gluten (whole grain flour)

DIRECTIONS

1. In a mixing bowl, combine grated sweet potato, eggs, onions, flax seeds, and whole grain flour. Mix well.
2. Heat a non-stick skillet over medium heat and add a little oil if necessary.
3. Spoon the mixture onto the skillet, forming small patties.
4. Cook for about 3-4 minutes on each side until golden brown and cooked through.
5. Serve warm.

Pancakes and Fritters

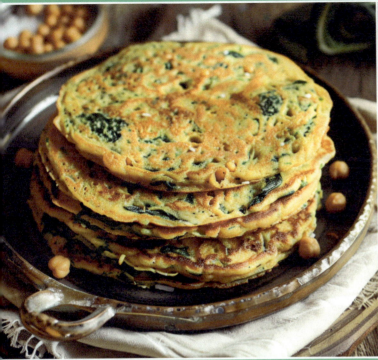

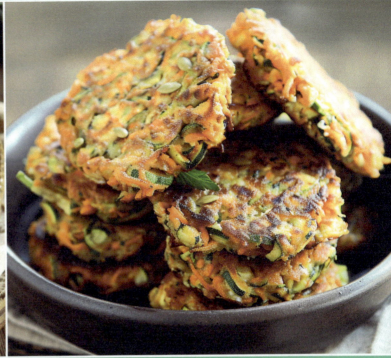

Spinach and Chickpea Pancakes

🍴 2 | ⏲ 75 min (plus soaking overnight) | Macronutrients (per serving): Calories: 240 | Protein: 10 g Fat: 4 g Carbs: 40 g

INGREDIENTS

- 1 cup whole grain flour
- 1 cup water
- 1/2 cup cooked chickpeas, mashed (prepare 1/4 cup dry chickpeas)
- 1 cup spinach, chopped
- 1/4 cup onions, finely diced

Allergens:
- Gluten (whole grain flour)

DIRECTIONS

1. Soak 1/4 cup of dry chickpeas in water overnight. Drain and rinse. Cook in boiling water for about 1 hour until tender. Drain and mash.
2. In a bowl, combine whole grain flour and water until smooth.
3. Stir in mashed chickpeas, chopped spinach, and diced onions.
4. Heat a non-stick skillet over medium heat. Pour 1/4 cup of batter for each pancake.
5. Cook until bubbles form, then flip and cook until golden brown, about 2-3 minutes per side.

Carrot and Zucchini Fritters

🍴 2 | ⏲ 20 min | Macronutrients (per serving): Calories: 240 | Protein: 10 g Fat: 8 g Carbs: 30 g

INGREDIENTS

- 1 carrot, grated
- 1 zucchini, grated
- 2 eggs
- 1/4 cup whole grain flour
- 2 tablespoons pumpkin seeds

Allergens:
- Eggs
- Gluten (whole grain flour)

DIRECTIONS

1. In a mixing bowl, combine grated carrot, grated zucchini, eggs, whole grain flour, and pumpkin seeds. Mix well.
2. Heat a non-stick skillet over medium heat and add a little oil if necessary.
3. Spoon the mixture onto the skillet, forming small patties.
4. Cook for about 3-4 minutes on each side until golden brown and cooked through.
5. Serve warm.

Crispy and Delicious Toasts

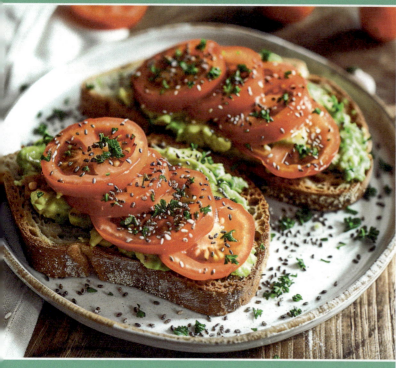 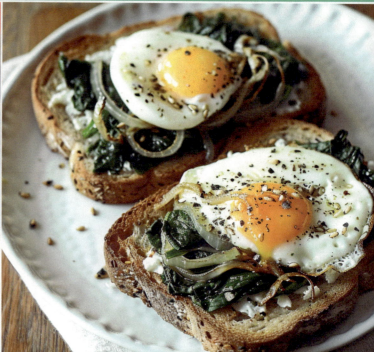

Avocado and Tomato Toast

🍴 2 | 🕐 10 min | Macronutrients (per serving): Calories: 300 | Protein: 8 g / Fat: 20 g / Carbs: 28 g

INGREDIENTS

- 2 slices whole grain bread
- 1 avocado
- 1 tomato, sliced
- 1 tablespoon chia seeds
- 1 garlic clove, minced

Allergens:
- Gluten (whole grain bread)

DIRECTIONS

1. Toast the whole grain bread slices until golden brown.
2. Mash the avocado and spread it evenly over the toast.
3. Top with sliced tomatoes.
4. Sprinkle with chia seeds and minced garlic.
5. Serve immediately.

Spinach and Egg Toast

🍴 2 | 🕐 15 min | Macronutrients (per serving): Calories: 350 | Protein: 14 g / Fat: 20 g / Carbs: 30 g

INGREDIENTS

- 2 slices whole grain bread
- 2 eggs
- 1 cup spinach, chopped
- 1/4 cup onions, finely diced
- 1 tablespoon olive oil (optional for cooking)

Allergens:
- Gluten (whole grain bread)
- Eggs

DIRECTIONS

1. Toast the whole grain bread slices until golden brown.
2. Heat olive oil in a skillet over medium heat.
3. Add onions and cook until translucent, about 3 minutes.
4. Add spinach and cook until wilted, about 2 minutes.
5. In the same skillet, cook the eggs to your preference (scrambled, fried, etc.).
6. Place the cooked spinach and onions on the toast, then top with eggs.

Crispy and Delicious Toasts

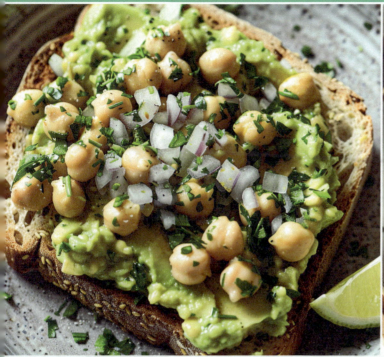

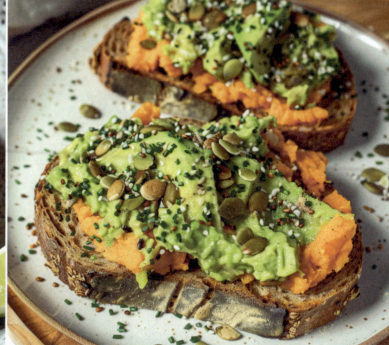

Chickpea and Avocado Toast

2 | 70 min (plus soaking overnight) | Macronutrients (per serving): Calories: 320 | Protein: 10 g Fat: 18 g Carbs: 36 g

INGREDIENTS

- 2 slices whole grain bread
- 1 avocado
- 1/2 cup cooked chickpeas, mashed
- 1/4 cup onions, finely diced
- 1 tablespoon lemon juice

Allergens:
- Gluten (whole grain bread)

DIRECTIONS

1. Soak 1/4 cup of dry chickpeas in water overnight. Drain and rinse. Cook chickpeas in boiling water for about 1 hour until tender. Drain and mash.
2. Toast the whole grain bread slices until golden brown.
3. Mash the avocado and chickpeas together in a bowl.
4. Stir in the diced onions and lemon juice.
5. Spread the chickpea and avocado mixture evenly over the toast.
6. Serve immediately.

Sweet Potato and Avocado Toast

2 | 20 min | Macronutrients (per serving): Calories: 340 | Protein: 8 g Fat: 18 g Carbs: 42 g

INGREDIENTS

- 2 slices whole grain bread
- 1 small sweet potato, cooked and mashed
- 1 avocado
- 1 tablespoon pumpkin seeds
- 1 garlic clove, minced

Allergens:
- Gluten (whole grain bread)

DIRECTIONS

1. Toast the whole grain bread slices until golden brown.
2. Mash the sweet potato and avocado together in a bowl.
3. Spread the sweet potato and avocado mixture evenly over the toast.
4. Sprinkle with pumpkin seeds and minced garlic.
5. Serve immediately.

Light Breakfasts with Fruits and Nuts

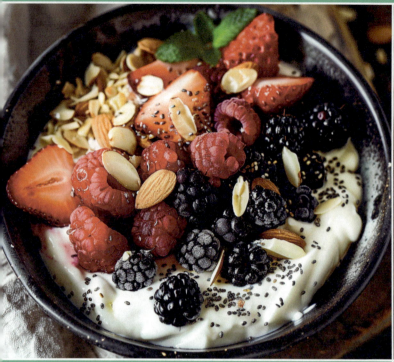
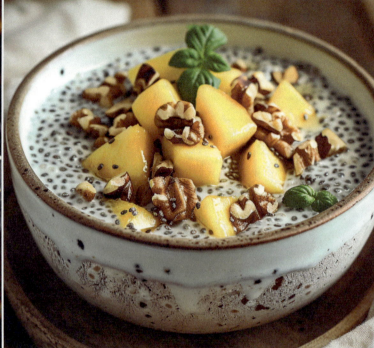

Greek Yogurt with Berries and Almonds

1 | 5 min | Macronutrients (per serving): Calories: 350 | Protein: 20 g Fat: 15 g Carbs: 35 g

INGREDIENTS

- 1 cup Greek yogurt
- 1/2 cup mixed berries (blueberries, raspberries, strawberries)
- 1/4 cup almonds, chopped
- 1 tablespoon chia seeds
- 1 tablespoon honey (optional)

Allergens:
- Dairy (Greek yogurt)
- Nuts (almonds)

DIRECTIONS

1. In a bowl, combine Greek yogurt and mixed berries.
2. Top with chopped almonds and chia seeds.
3. Drizzle with honey if desired.
4. Serve immediately.

Chia Pudding with Mango and Walnuts

1 | 35 min | Macronutrients (per serving): Calories: 300 | Protein: 8 g Fat: 20 g Carbs: 25 g

INGREDIENTS

- 1/4 cup chia seeds
- 1 cup almond milk
- 1/2 mango, diced
- 1/4 cup walnuts, chopped
- 1 tablespoon maple syrup (optional)

Allergens:
- Nuts (almond milk, walnuts)

DIRECTIONS

1. In a bowl, combine chia seeds and almond milk. Stir well and let sit for at least 30 minutes or overnight in the refrigerator.
2. Once the chia pudding is set, top with diced mango and chopped walnuts.
3. Drizzle with maple syrup if desired.
4. Serve chilled.

Light Breakfasts with Fruits and Nuts

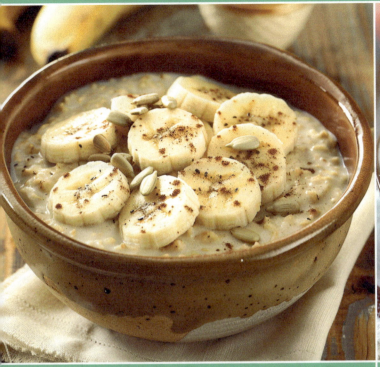

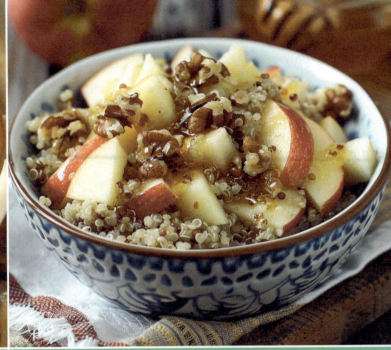

Oatmeal with Bananas and Sunflower Seeds

🍴 2 | 🕐 12 min | Macronutrients (per serving): Calories: 350 | Protein: 10 g | Fat: 12 g | Carbs: 55 g

INGREDIENTS

- 1 cup oats
- 2 cups water or almond milk
- 1 banana, sliced
- 2 tablespoons sunflower seeds
- 1 teaspoon cinnamon (optional)

Allergens:
- Nuts (almond milk, if used)

DIRECTIONS

1. In a medium saucepan, bring water or almond milk to a boil.
2. Add oats and reduce heat to a simmer. Cook for about 5-7 minutes, or until the oats are tender.
3. Stir in sliced banana and sunflower seeds.
4. Sprinkle with cinnamon if desired.
5. Serve warm.

Quinoa Breakfast Bowl with Apples and Flax Seeds

🍴 2 | 🕐 25 min | Macronutrients (per serving): Calories: 400 | Protein: 12 g | Fat: 16 g | Carbs: 50 g

INGREDIENTS

- 1 cup quinoa, cooked
- 1 apple, diced
- 2 tablespoons flax seeds
- 1/4 cup walnuts, chopped
- 1 tablespoon honey (optional)

Allergens:
- Nuts (walnuts)

DIRECTIONS

1. Cook quinoa according to package instructions (on average 15-20 minutes).
2. Combine cooked quinoa, diced apple, flax seeds, and chopped walnuts in a bowl.
3. Drizzle with honey if desired.
4. Serve warm or chilled.

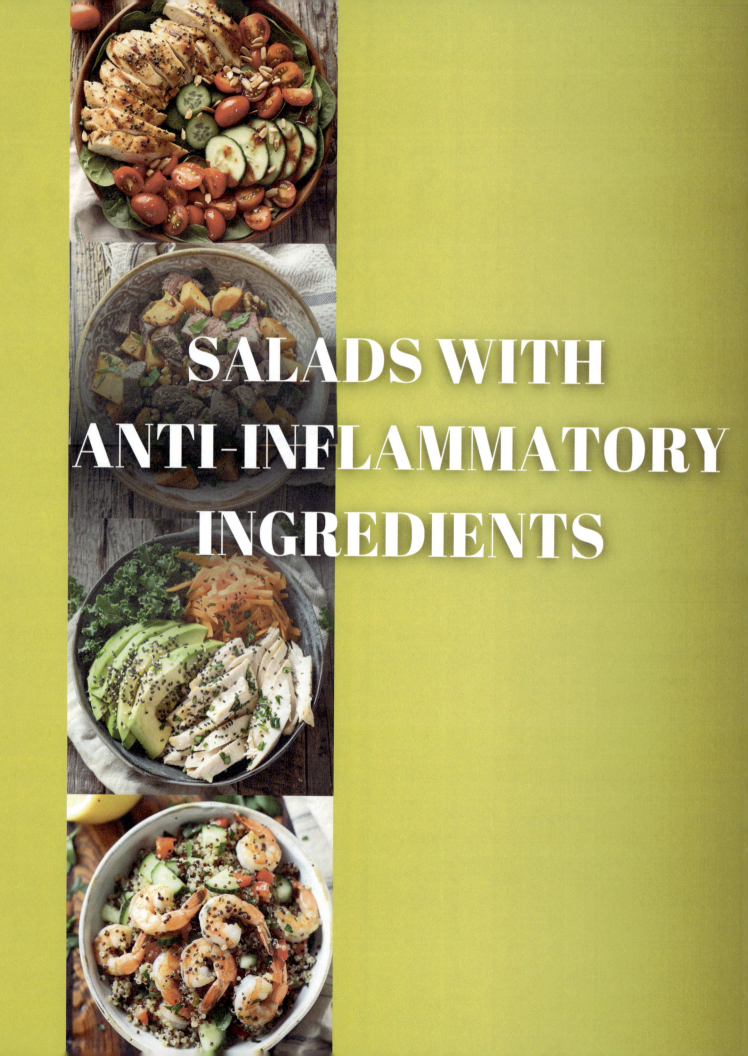

SALADS WITH ANTI-INFLAMMATORY INGREDIENTS

Salads with Meat

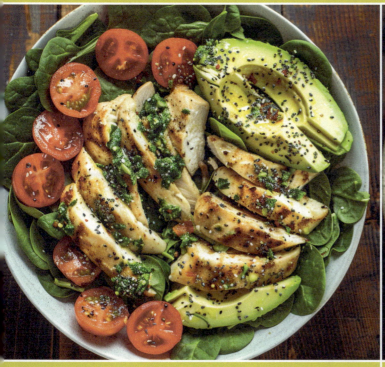 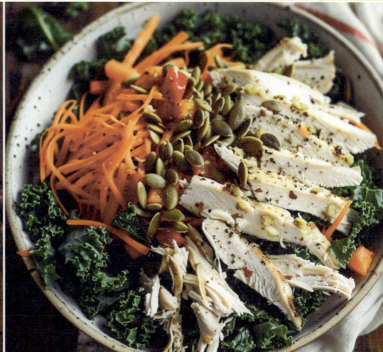

Chicken and Avocado Salad

| 2 | 30 min | Macronutrients (per serving): Calories: 350 | Protein: 25 g Fat: 22 g Carbs: 10 g |

INGREDIENTS

- 1 cup cooked chicken breast, diced
- 1 avocado, diced
- 1 cup spinach, chopped
- 1/2 cup cherry tomatoes, halved
- 1 tablespoon chia seeds

Allergens:
- None

DIRECTIONS

1. Boil the chicken breast for 15-20 minutes and let it cool slightly.
2. Combine diced chicken breast, diced avocado, chopped spinach, and halved cherry tomatoes in a large bowl.
3. Sprinkle with chia seeds.
4. Toss gently to mix.
5. Serve immediately.

Turkey and Kale Salad

| 2 | 30 min | Macronutrients (per serving): Calories: 320 | Protein: 30 g Fat: 15 g Carbs: 15 g |

INGREDIENTS

- 1 cup cooked turkey breast, sliced
- 2 cups kale, chopped
- 1/2 cup shredded carrots
- 1/4 cup pumpkin seeds
- 1/4 cup red bell pepper, diced

Allergens:
- None

DIRECTIONS

1. Boil the turkey breast for 20-25 minutes and let it cool slightly
2. Combine sliced turkey breast, chopped kale, shredded carrots, and diced red bell pepper in a large bowl.
3. Sprinkle with pumpkin seeds.
4. Toss gently to mix.
5. Serve immediately.

Salads with Meat

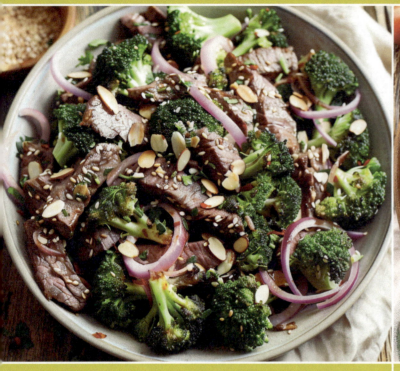

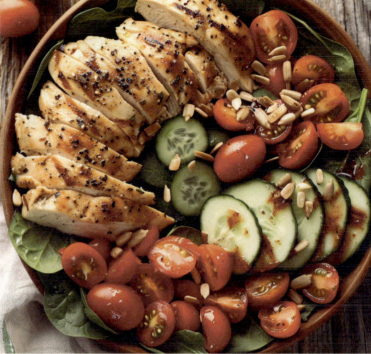

Beef and Broccoli Salad

🍴 2 ⏱ 30 min Macronutrients (per serving): Calories: 400 Protein: 28 g Fat: 25 g Carbs: 12 g

INGREDIENTS

- 1 cup cooked grass-fed beef, sliced
- 1 cup broccoli florets, steamed
- 1/2 cup red onion, thinly sliced
- 1/4 cup almonds, sliced
- 1 tablespoon flax seeds

Allergens:
- Nuts (almonds)

DIRECTIONS

1. Simmer the beef slices for 15-20 minutes and let it cool slightly.
2. Steam the broccoli for 5-7 minutes.
3. In a large bowl, combine sliced beef, steamed broccoli florets, and thinly sliced red onion.
4. Sprinkle with sliced almonds and flax seeds.
5. Toss gently to mix.
6. Serve immediately.

Chicken and Spinach Salad

🍴 2 ⏱ 30 min Macronutrients (per serving): Calories: 350 Protein: 25 g Fat: 20 g Carbs: 12 g

INGREDIENTS

- 1 cup cooked chicken breast, diced
- 2 cups spinach, chopped
- 1/2 cup cucumbers, diced
- 1/4 cup sunflower seeds
- 1/2 cup cherry tomatoes, halved

Allergens:
- Seeds (sunflower seeds)

DIRECTIONS

1. Boil the chicken breast for 15-20 minutes and let it cool slightly.
2. Combine diced chicken breast, chopped spinach, diced cucumbers, and halved cherry tomatoes in a large bowl.
3. Sprinkle with sunflower seeds.
4. Toss gently to mix.
5. Serve immediately.

Salads with Meat

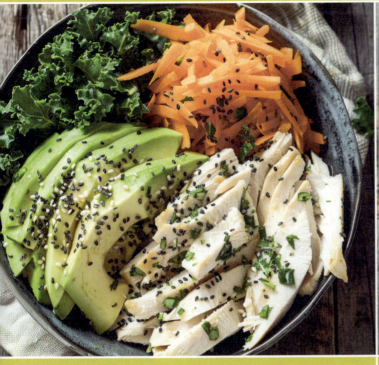
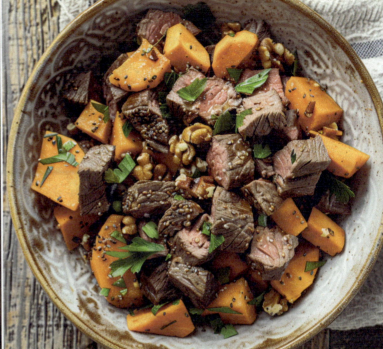

Turkey and Avocado Salad

2	30 min	Macronutrients (per serving): Calories: 350	Protein: 30 g Fat: 22 g Carbs: 10 g

INGREDIENTS

- 1 cup cooked turkey breast, sliced
- 1 avocado, diced
- 1 cup kale, chopped
- 1/2 cup shredded carrots
- 1 tablespoon chia seeds

Allergens:
- None

DIRECTIONS

1. Boil the turkey breast for 20-25 minutes and let it cool slightly
2. Combine sliced turkey breast, diced avocado, chopped kale, and shredded carrots in a large bowl.
3. Sprinkle with chia seeds.
4. Toss gently to mix.
5. Serve immediately.

Beef and Sweet Potato Salad

2	30 min	Macronutrients (per serving): Calories: 400	Protein: 28 g Fat: 20 g Carbs: 25 g

INGREDIENTS

- 1 cup cooked grass-fed beef, sliced
- 1 cup sweet potato, cooked and diced
- 1/2 cup red bell pepper, diced
- 1/4 cup walnuts, chopped
- 1 tablespoon flax seeds

Allergens:
- Nuts (walnuts)

DIRECTIONS

1. Boil the sweet potatoes for 15-20 minutes until tender, and let it cool slightly.
2. Pan-fry the beef slices in refined coconut oil for 4-5 minutes and let them cool slightly.
3. In a large bowl, combine sliced beef, cooked and diced sweet potato, and diced red bell pepper.
4. Sprinkle with chopped walnuts and flax seeds.
5. Toss gently to mix.
6. Serve immediately.

Salads with Seafood

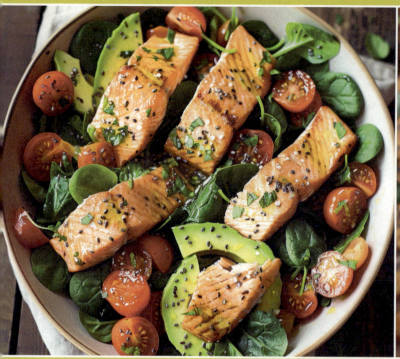

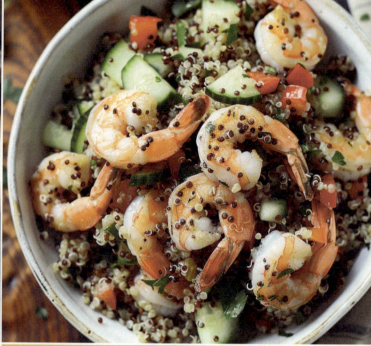

Salmon and Avocado Salad

| 2 | 30 min | Macronutrients (per serving):
Calories: 400 | Protein: 28 g
Fat: 30 g
Carbs: 10 g |

INGREDIENTS

- 1 cup cooked salmon, flaked
- 1 avocado, diced
- 1 cup spinach, chopped
- 1/2 cup cherry tomatoes, halved
- 1 tablespoon chia seeds
- 1 tablespoon olive oil, salt

Allergens:
- Fish (salmon)

DIRECTIONS

1. Bake the salmon in the oven with a drizzle of olive oil and a sprinkle of salt for 15-20 minutes.
2. Combine flaked salmon, diced avocado, chopped spinach, and halved cherry tomatoes in a large bowl.
3. Sprinkle with chia seeds.
4. Toss gently to mix.
5. Serve immediately.

Shrimp and Quinoa Salad

| 2 | 30 min | Macronutrients (per serving):
Calories: 350 | Protein: 25 g
Fat: 10 g
Carbs: 35 g |

INGREDIENTS

- 1 cup cooked shrimp
- 1 cup cooked quinoa
- 1/2 cup cucumbers, diced
- 1/4 cup red bell pepper, diced
- 1 tablespoon flax seeds
- 1/2 lemon, halved (optional)
- 1 clove garlic, smashed (optional)
- Salt, to taste

Allergens:
- Shrimp

DIRECTIONS

1. Boil the shrimp with salt, lemon (optional), and garlic (optional) for 2-3 minutes until they turn pink and opaque. Transfer them to a bowl of ice water to cool, then dry and chop.
2. Cook quinoa according to package instructions (on average, 15-20 minutes).
3. Combine cooked shrimp, quinoa, diced cucumbers, and red bell pepper in a large bowl.
4. Sprinkle with flax seeds.
5. Toss gently to mix.

Salads with Seafood

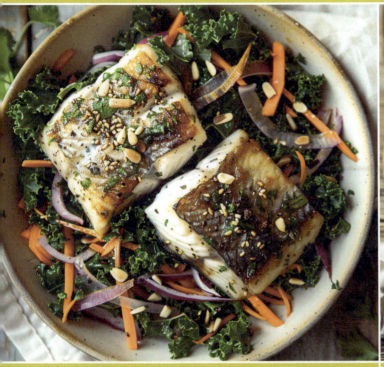

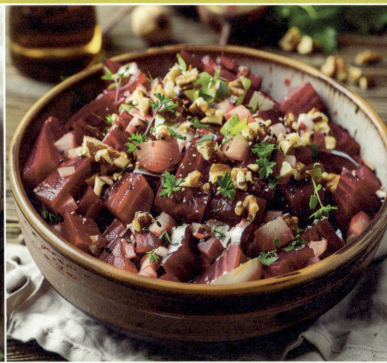

Mackerel and Kale Salad

2 | 30 min | Macronutrients (per serving): Calories: 370 | Protein: 30 g Fat: 25 g Carbs: 15 g

INGREDIENTS

- 1 cup cooked mackerel, flaked
- 2 cups kale, chopped
- 1/2 cup shredded carrots
- 1/4 cup sunflower seeds
- 1/4 cup red onion, thinly sliced
- 1 tablespoon olive oil
- Salt and pepper to taste

Allergens:
- Fish (mackerel), Seeds (sunflower seeds)

DIRECTIONS

1. Preheat the oven to 375°F (190°C); place the mackerel fillet on a baking sheet, drizzle with olive oil, season with salt and pepper, and bake for 15-20 minutes until the fish flakes easily with a fork.
2. Combine flaked mackerel, chopped kale, shredded carrots, and thinly sliced red onion in a large bowl.
3. Sprinkle with sunflower seeds.
4. Toss gently to mix.
5. Serve immediately.

Herring and Beet Salad

2 | 45 min | Macronutrients (per serving): Calories: 380 | Protein: 22 g Fat: 28 g Carbs: 18 g

INGREDIENTS

- 1 cup cooked herring, flaked
- 1 cup cooked beets, diced
- 1/2 cup diced cucumber
- 1/4 cup walnuts, chopped
- 1 tablespoon pumpkin seeds
- 1 tablespoon olive oil
- Salt and pepper to taste

Allergens:
- Herring
- Walnuts
- Pumpkin seeds

DIRECTIONS

1. Boil or steam beets for 30-40 minutes until tender, cool, peel, and dice to make 1 cup for the salad.
2. Bake a herring fillet seasoned with salt and pepper at 375°F (190°C) for 15-20 minutes, cool, and flake with a fork to make 1 cup.
3. In a large bowl, combine diced beets, diced cucumber, and flaked herring.
4. Drizzle with olive oil, sprinkle with chopped walnuts and pumpkin seeds.
5. Toss gently, season with salt and pepper to taste, and serve immediately.

Salads with Seafood

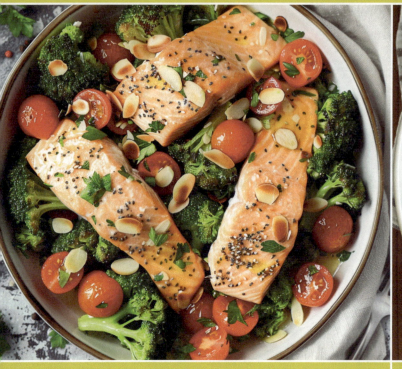

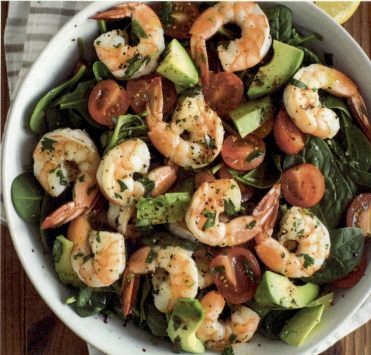

Salmon and Broccoli Salad

🍴 2 | ⏱ 30 min | Macronutrients (per serving): Calories: 400 | Protein: 28 g Fat: 30 g Carbs: 10 g

INGREDIENTS

- 1 cup cooked salmon, flaked
- 1 cup steamed broccoli florets
- 1/2 cup cherry tomatoes, halved
- 1/4 cup almonds, sliced
- 1 tablespoon chia seeds
- 1 tablespoon olive oil (optional)
- Salt and pepper to taste

Allergens:
- Salmon
- Almonds

DIRECTIONS

1. Preheat the oven to 375°F (190°C). Place the salmon fillet on a baking sheet, drizzle with olive oil, season with salt and pepper, and bake for 15-20 minutes until it flakes easily. Let it cool and flake the salmon.
2. Steam broccoli florets for 5-7 minutes until tender.
3. In a large bowl, combine flaked salmon, steamed broccoli, and halved cherry tomatoes.
4. Sprinkle with sliced almonds and chia seeds.
5. Drizzle with olive oil if desired, season with salt and pepper, and toss gently. Serve immediately.

Shrimp and Avocado Salad

🍴 2 | ⏱ 15 min | Macronutrients (per serving): Calories: 380 | Protein: 25 g Fat: 25 g Carbs: 12 g

INGREDIENTS

- 1 avocado, diced
- 1 cup spinach, chopped
- 1 cup cooked shrimp, peeled and deveined
- 1/2 cup cherry tomatoes, halved
- 1 tablespoon flax seeds
- 1 tablespoon olive oil (optional)
- Salt and pepper to taste

Allergens:
- Shrimp

DIRECTIONS

1. Boil the shrimp with salt, lemon, and garlic (optional) for 2-3 minutes until they turn pink and opaque. Transfer them to a bowl of ice water to cool, then drain and pat dry.
2. In a large bowl, combine cooked shrimp, diced avocado, chopped spinach, and halved cherry tomatoes.
3. Sprinkle with flax seeds.
4. Drizzle with olive oil if using, season with salt and pepper to taste, and toss gently to mix.
5. Serve immediately.

Vegetarian & Vegan Salads

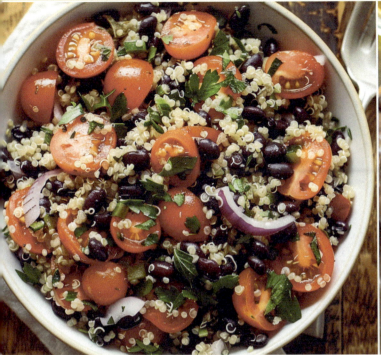

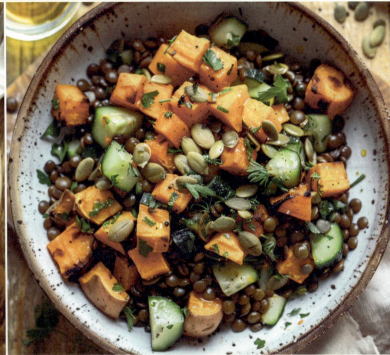

Quinoa and Black Bean Salad

Serves: 2 | Time: 25 min

Macronutrients (per serving):
Calories: 350 | Protein: 12 g | Fat: 12 g | Carbs: 50 g

INGREDIENTS

- 1 cup cooked quinoa
- 1 cup black beans, rinsed and drained
- 1/2 cup cherry tomatoes, halved
- 1/2 cup diced red bell pepper
- 1/4 cup chopped red onion
- 2 tablespoons sunflower seeds
- 1 tablespoon olive oil
- Salt and pepper to taste

Allergens:
- Sunflower seeds

DIRECTIONS

1. Rinse 1/2 cup quinoa under cold water. Combine with 1 cup water in a pot, boil, then reduce heat and simmer for 15 minutes or until water is absorbed. Let cool.
2. While cooking, rinse and drain 1 cup black beans. Halve cherry tomatoes, dice red bell pepper, and chop red onion.
3. In a large bowl, combine cooked quinoa, black beans, tomatoes, bell pepper, and onion.
4. Sprinkle with sunflower seeds, drizzle with olive oil, and season with salt and pepper. Toss gently and serve immediately.

Lentil and Roasted Vegetable Salad

Serves: 2 | Time: 40 min

Macronutrients (per serving):
Calories: 400 | Protein: 15 g | Fat: 14 g | Carbs: 12 g

INGREDIENTS

- 1 cup cooked lentils
- 1 cup roasted sweet potatoes
- 1/2 cup roasted carrots, diced
- 1/2 cup diced cucumber
- 1/4 cup pumpkin seeds
- 1 tablespoon olive oil
- Salt and pepper to taste

Allergens:
- Pumpkin seeds

DIRECTIONS

1. Rinse 1/2 cup of lentils under cold water. Combine with 1 cup of water in a pot, boil, reduce heat, and simmer for 20-25 minutes until tender. Drain and let cool.
2. Preheat the oven to 400°F (200°C). Peel and dice sweet potatoes and carrots, toss with olive oil, salt, and pepper. Roast for 25-30 minutes until tender, then cool.
3. Dice the cucumber.
4. In a large bowl, combine lentils, roasted sweet potatoes, carrots, and cucumber.
5. Sprinkle with pumpkin seeds, drizzle with olive oil, season with salt and pepper, and toss gently to mix.

Vegetarian & Vegan Salads

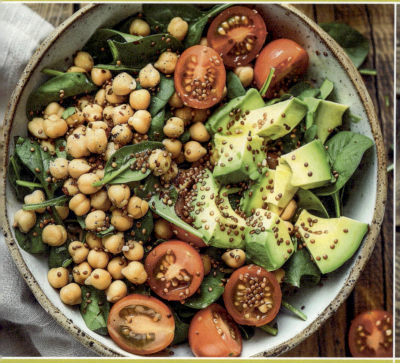

Chickpea and Avocado Salad

- 2
- 65 min
- Macronutrients (per serving):
  Calories: 380
- Protein: 12 g
  Fat: 25 g
  Carbs: 30 g

INGREDIENTS

- 1 cup cooked chickpeas, rinsed and drained
- 1 avocado, diced
- 1 cup spinach, chopped
- 1/2 cup cherry tomatoes, halved
- 1 tablespoon flax seeds
- 1 tablespoon olive oil
- Salt and pepper to taste

Allergens:
- None

DIRECTIONS

1. Rinse 1/2 cup of dried chickpeas under cold water. Place in a pot with 2 cups of water and boil. Reduce heat and simmer for 45-60 minutes until tender. Drain and let cool.
2. Rinse and drain 1 cup of cooked chickpeas. Dice the avocado, chop the spinach, and halve the cherry tomatoes.
3. In a large bowl, combine chickpeas, diced avocado, chopped spinach, and halved cherry tomatoes.
4. Sprinkle with flax seeds, drizzle with olive oil, and season with salt and pepper to taste.
5. Toss gently to mix and serve immediately.

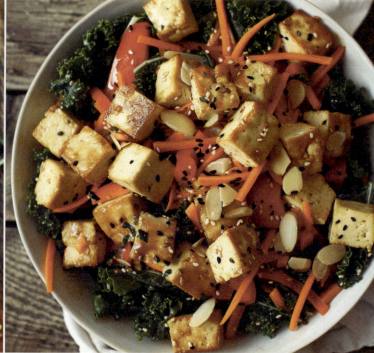

Tofu and Kale Salad

- 2
- 20 min
- Macronutrients (per serving):
  Calories: 350
- Protein: 14 g
  Fat: 22 g
  Carbs: 20 g

INGREDIENTS

- 1 cup firm tofu, cubed
- 2 cups kale, chopped
- 1/2 cup shredded carrots
- 1/2 cup diced red bell pepper
- 2 tablespoons chopped almonds
- 1 tablespoon olive oil
- Salt and pepper to taste

Allergens:
- Nuts (almonds)

DIRECTIONS

1. Press and drain tofu to remove excess water. Cut into cubes.
2. Heat a skillet over medium heat, add olive oil, and cook tofu cubes for 5-7 minutes until golden brown. Let cool.
3. Chop the kale, shred the carrots, and dice the red bell pepper.
4. In a large bowl, combine cooked tofu, chopped kale, shredded carrots, and diced red bell pepper.
5. Sprinkle with chopped almonds, drizzle with olive oil, and season with salt and pepper to taste.
6. Toss gently to mix and serve immediately.

Vegetarian & Vegan Salads

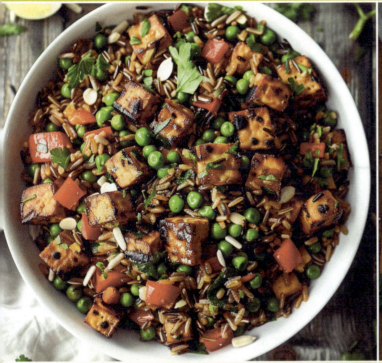

Tempeh and Wild Rice Salad

| 2 | 55 min | Macronutrients (per serving): Calories: 400 | Protein: 18 g Fat: 14 g Carbs: 50 g |

INGREDIENTS

- 1 cup tempeh, cubed
- 1 cup cooked wild rice
- 1/2 cup green peas
- 1/2 cup diced red bell pepper
- 1 tablespoon sunflower seeds
- 1 tablespoon olive oil
- Salt and pepper to taste

Allergens:
- Tempeh
- Sunflower seeds

DIRECTIONS

1. Rinse 1/2 cup wild rice under cold water. Combine with 1 1/2 cups water in a pot, boil, reduce heat, and simmer for 40-45 minutes until tender. Drain and cool.
2. Heat olive oil in a skillet over medium heat. Add cubed tempeh and cook for 5-7 minutes until golden brown. Let cool.
3. Thaw green peas if frozen and dice red bell pepper.
4. In a large bowl, combine cooked wild rice, tempeh, green peas, and red bell pepper.
5. Sprinkle with sunflower seeds, drizzle with olive oil, and season with salt and pepper.
6. Toss gently to mix and serve immediately.

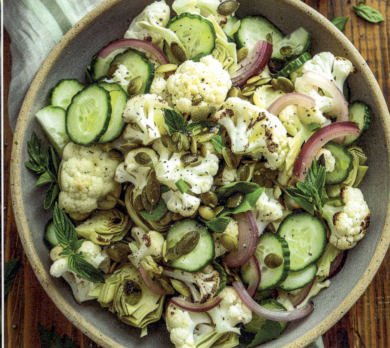

Cauliflower and Artichoke Salad

| 2 | 12 min | Macronutrients (per serving): Calories: 220 | Protein: 6 g Fat: 14 g Carbs: 20 g |

INGREDIENTS

- 1 cup cauliflower florets
- 1 cup artichoke hearts
- 1/2 cup diced cucumbers
- 1/4 cup diced red onion
- 1 tablespoon pumpkin seeds
- 1 tablespoon olive oil
- Salt and pepper to taste

Allergens:
- Pumpkin seeds

DIRECTIONS

1. Steam cauliflower florets for 5-7 minutes until tender. Let cool.
2. While the cauliflower is steaming, chop the artichoke hearts, dice the cucumbers, and dice the red onion.
3. In a large bowl, combine steamed cauliflower, chopped artichoke hearts, diced cucumbers, and diced red onion.
4. Sprinkle with pumpkin seeds, drizzle with olive oil, and season with salt and pepper to taste.
5. Toss gently to mix and serve immediately.

Vegetarian & Vegan Salads

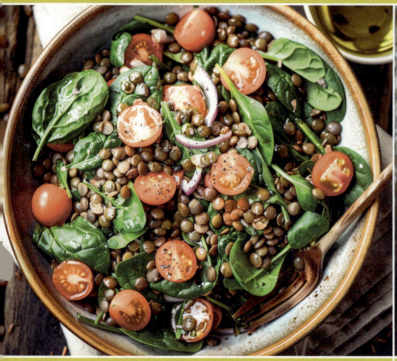

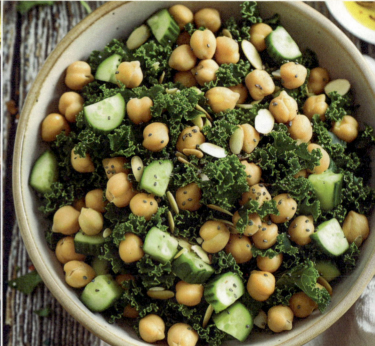

Lentil and Spinach Salad

Serves: 2 | Time: 30 min

Macronutrients (per serving):
Calories: 300
Protein: 15 g
Fat: 10 g
Carbs: 35 g

INGREDIENTS

- 1 cup cooked lentils
- 1 cup spinach, chopped
- 1/2 cup cherry tomatoes, halved
- 1/4 cup red onion, diced
- 1 tablespoon flax seeds
- 1 tablespoon olive oil
- Salt and pepper to taste

Allergens:
- None

DIRECTIONS

1. Rinse 1/2 cup of lentils under cold water. Combine with 1 cup of water in a pot, boil, then reduce heat and simmer for 20-25 minutes until tender. Drain and let cool.
2. While the lentils are cooking, chop the spinach, halve the cherry tomatoes, and dice the red onion.
3. In a large bowl, combine cooked lentils, chopped spinach, cherry tomatoes, and red onion.
4. Sprinkle with flax seeds, drizzle with olive oil, and season with salt and pepper to taste.
5. Toss gently to mix and serve immediately.

Chickpea and Kale Salad

Serves: 2 | Time: 65 min

Macronutrients (per serving):
Calories: 350
Protein: 14 g
Fat: 18 g
Carbs: 40 g

INGREDIENTS

- 1 cup cooked chickpeas
- 2 cups kale, chopped
- 1/2 cup diced cucumber
- 1/4 cup almonds, chopped
- 1 tablespoon chia seeds
- 1 tablespoon olive oil
- Salt and pepper to taste

Allergens:
- Almonds

DIRECTIONS

1. Rinse 1/2 cup of dried chickpeas under cold water. Place in a pot with 2 cups of water and boil. Reduce heat and simmer for 45-60 minutes until tender. Drain and let cool.
2. While the chickpeas are cooking, chop the kale and dice the cucumber.
3. In a large bowl, combine cooked chickpeas, chopped kale, and diced cucumber.
4. Sprinkle with chopped almonds and chia seeds.
5. Drizzle with olive oil, season with salt and pepper to taste, and toss gently to mix. Serve immediately.

Vegetarian & Vegan Salads

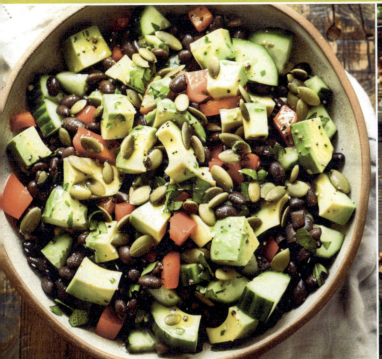

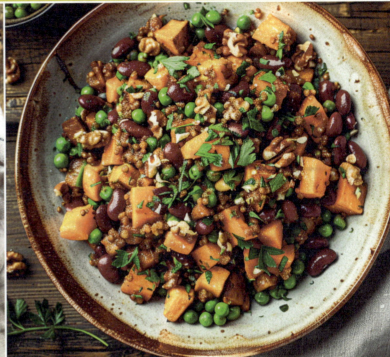

Black Bean and Avocado Salad

		Macronutrients (per serving):	Protein: 12 g
2	65 min	Calories: 380	Fat: 20 g Carbs: 40 g

INGREDIENTS

- 1 cup cooked black beans
- 1 avocado, diced
- 1/2 cup diced red bell pepper
- 1/2 cup diced cucumber
- 1 tablespoon pumpkin seeds
- 1 tablespoon olive oil
- Salt and pepper to taste

Allergens:
- None

DIRECTIONS

1. Rinse 1/2 cup of dried black beans under cold water. Place in a pot with 2 cups of water and bring to a boil. Reduce heat and simmer for 45-60 minutes until tender. Drain and let cool.
2. While the black beans are cooking, dice the avocado, red bell pepper, and cucumber.
3. In a large bowl, combine cooked black beans, diced avocado, red bell pepper, and cucumber.
4. Sprinkle with pumpkin seeds, drizzle with olive oil and season with salt and pepper to taste.
5. Toss gently to mix and serve immediately.

Red Bean and Sweet Potato Salad

		Macronutrients (per serving):	Protein: 14 g
2	90 min	Calories: 400	Fat: 18 g Carbs: 50 g

INGREDIENTS

- 1 cup cooked red beans
- 1 cup roasted sweet potatoes
- 1/2 cup green peas
- 1/4 cup walnuts, chopped
- 1 tablespoon olive oil
- Salt and pepper to taste

Allergens:
- Nuts (walnuts)

DIRECTIONS

1. Rinse 1/2 cup of dried red beans under cold water. Place in a pot with 2 cups of water, bring to a boil, reduce heat, and simmer for 45-60 minutes until tender. Drain and let cool.
2. Preheat the oven to 400°F (200°C). Peel and dice the sweet potatoes, toss with olive oil, salt, and pepper, and roast for 25-30 minutes until tender. Let cool. Thaw the green peas if frozen.
3. In a large bowl, combine cooked red beans, roasted sweet potatoes, and green peas.
4. Sprinkle with chopped walnuts, drizzle with olive oil, and season with salt and pepper. Toss gently to mix and serve immediately.

Vegetarian & Vegan Salads

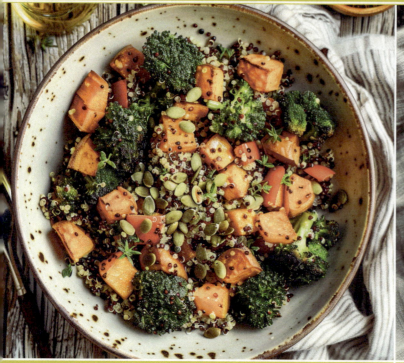

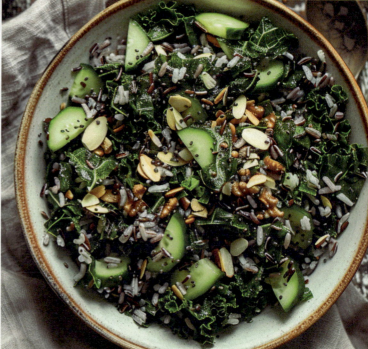

Quinoa and Roasted Vegetable Salad

🍴 2 | 🕐 45 min | Macronutrients (per serving): Calories: 350 | Protein: 10 g Fat: 14 g Carbs: 45 g

INGREDIENTS

- 1 cup cooked quinoa
- 1 cup roasted broccoli florets
- 1 cup roasted sweet potatoes
- 1/2 cup diced red bell pepper
- 1 tablespoon pumpkin seeds
- 1 tablespoon olive oil
- Salt and pepper to taste

Allergens:
- Pumpkin seeds

DIRECTIONS

1. Rinse 1/2 cup of quinoa under cold water. Combine with 1 cup of water in a pot, bring to a boil, reduce heat, and simmer for 15 minutes until water is absorbed. Let cool.
2. Preheat the oven to 400°F (200°C). Toss broccoli florets and diced sweet potatoes with olive oil, salt, and pepper. Roast on a baking sheet for 20-25 minutes until tender. Let cool.
3. Dice the red bell pepper.
4. Combine cooked quinoa, roasted broccoli, sweet potatoes, and red bell pepper in a large bowl.
5. Sprinkle with pumpkin seeds, drizzle with olive oil, season with salt and pepper, and toss gently to mix.

Wild Rice and Kale Salad

🍴 2 | 🕐 50 min | Macronutrients (per serving): Calories: 400 | Protein: 12 g Fat: 18 g Carbs: 50 g

INGREDIENTS

- 1 cup cooked wild rice
- 2 cups kale, chopped
- 1/2 cup diced cucumber
- 1/4 cup chopped almonds
- 1 tablespoon chia seeds
- 1 tablespoon olive oil
- Salt and pepper to taste

Allergens:
- Nuts (almonds)
- Chia seeds

DIRECTIONS

1. Rinse 1/2 cup of wild rice under cold water. Combine with 1 1/2 cups of water in a pot, bring to a boil, then reduce heat and simmer for 40-45 minutes until tender. Drain and let cool.
2. While the wild rice is cooking, chop the kale and dice the cucumber.
3. Combine cooked wild rice, chopped kale, and diced cucumber in a large bowl.
4. Sprinkle with chopped almonds and chia seeds.
5. Drizzle with olive oil, season with salt and pepper to taste, and toss gently to mix.
6. Serve immediately.

Vegetarian & Vegan Salads

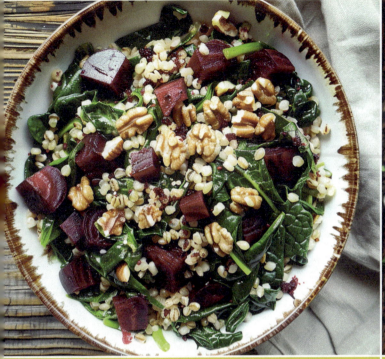

Barley and Beet Salad

Serves: 2 | Time: 75 min
Macronutrients (per serving):
Calories: 420 | Protein: 12 g | Fat: 20 g | Carbs: 50 g

INGREDIENTS

- 1 cup cooked barley
- 1 cup cooked beets, diced
- 1/2 cup spinach, chopped
- 1/4 cup walnuts, chopped
- 1 tablespoon flax seeds
- 1 tablespoon olive oil
- Salt and pepper to taste

Allergens:
- Nuts (walnuts)
- Flax seeds

DIRECTIONS

1. Rinse 1/2 cup of barley under cold water. Combine with 1 1/2 cups of water in a pot, bring to a boil, then reduce heat and simmer for 25-30 minutes until tender. Drain and let cool.
2. Boil or steam beets for 30-40 minutes until tender, let them cool, then peel and dice to make 1 cup of cooked beets.
3. Chop the spinach.
4. In a large bowl, combine cooked barley, diced beets, and chopped spinach.
5. Sprinkle with chopped walnuts and flax seeds.
6. Drizzle with olive oil, season with salt and pepper to taste, and toss gently to mix. Serve immediately.

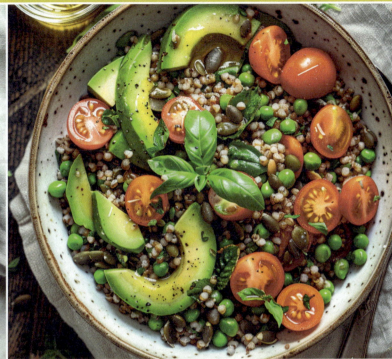

Buckwheat and Avocado Salad

Serves: 2 | Time: 25 min
Macronutrients (per serving):
Calories: 360 | Protein: 10 g | Fat: 18 g | Carbs: 40 g

INGREDIENTS

- 1 cup cooked buckwheat
- 1 avocado, diced
- 1/2 cup cherry tomatoes, halved
- 1/2 cup green peas
- 1 tablespoon sunflower seeds
- 1 tablespoon olive oil
- Salt and pepper to taste

Allergens:
- Sunflower seeds

DIRECTIONS

1. Rinse 1/2 cup of buckwheat under cold water. Combine with 1 cup of water in a pot, bring to a boil, then reduce heat and simmer for 15-20 minutes until tender. Drain and let cool.
2. Dice the avocado, halve the cherry tomatoes, and thaw the green peas if frozen.
3. In a large bowl, combine cooked buckwheat, diced avocado, cherry tomatoes, and green peas.
4. Sprinkle with sunflower seeds, drizzle with olive oil and season with salt and pepper to taste.
5. Toss gently to mix and serve immediately.

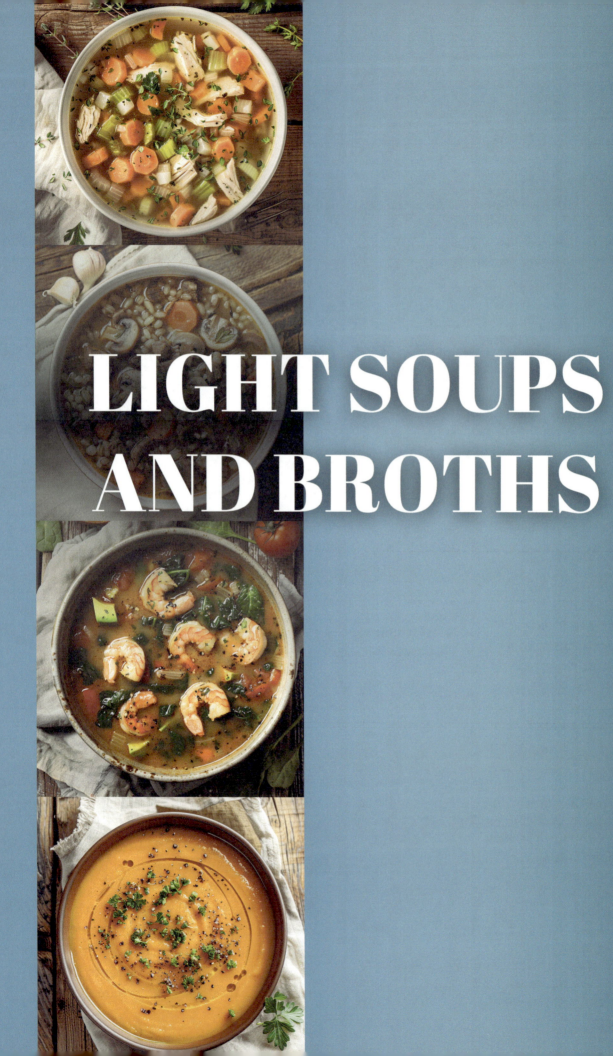

LIGHT SOUPS AND BROTHS

Meat Broths and Light Soups

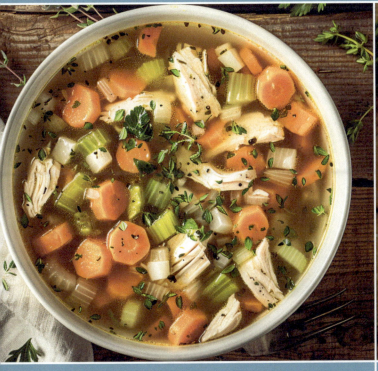

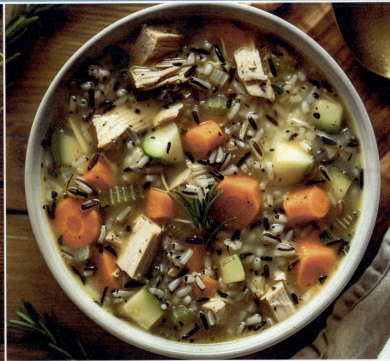

Chicken and Vegetable Broth

🍴 4 ⏲ 30 min Macronutrients (per serving): Protein: 20 g Fat: 10 g Calories: 250 Carbs: 15 g

INGREDIENTS

- 1 cup cooked chicken breast, shredded
- 2 carrots, sliced
- 2 celery stalks, sliced
- 1 onion, diced
- 3 cloves garlic, minced
- 4 cups chicken broth
- 1 tablespoon olive oil
- 1 teaspoon turmeric
- Salt and pepper to taste

Allergens:
- None

DIRECTIONS

1. Dice the onion, slice the carrots and celery, and mince the garlic.
2. Heat olive oil in a large pot over medium heat. Add the onion, carrots, and celery, and sauté for 5-7 minutes until the vegetables are softened. Add the garlic and cook for another minute.
3. Add the chicken broth, shredded chicken, and turmeric to the pot. Bring to a boil, then reduce the heat and simmer for 20 minutes. Season with salt and pepper to taste.
4. Serve hot.

Turkey and Wild Rice Soup

🍴 4 ⏲ 60 min Macronutrients (per serving): Protein: 18 g Fat: 10 g Calories: 300 Carbs: 35 g

INGREDIENTS

- 1 cup cooked turkey breast
- 1/2 cup wild rice
- 1 cup diced zucchini
- 1 cup diced carrots
- 1 onion, diced
- 3 cloves garlic, minced
- 4 cups turkey broth
- 1 tablespoon olive oil
- 1 teaspoon ginger
- Salt and pepper to taste

Allergens:
- None

DIRECTIONS

1. Rinse 1/2 cup wild rice under cold water. Combine with 1 1/2 cups water in a pot, bring to a boil, then simmer for 40 minutes until tender. Drain and set aside.
2. Dice the onion, carrots, zucchini, and mince the garlic. Heat olive oil in a pot over medium heat. Sauté the onion, carrots, and zucchini for 5-7 minutes until softened.
3. Add garlic and ginger, and cook for another minute. Add turkey broth, diced turkey, and cooked wild rice. Bring to a boil, then simmer for 20 minutes.
4. Season with salt and pepper. Serve hot.

Meat Broths and Light Soups

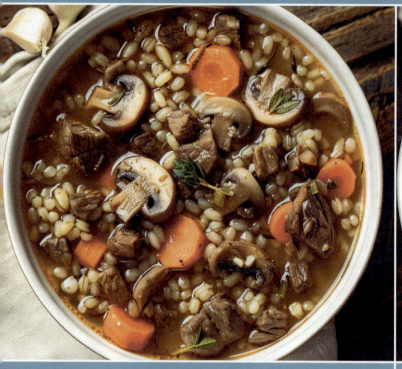
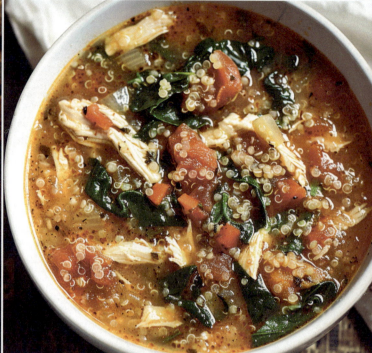

Beef and Barley Soup

Serves: 4 | Time: 60 min

Macronutrients (per serving):
Calories: 350
Protein: 20 g
Fat: 15 g
Carbs: 35 g

INGREDIENTS

- 1 cup cooked grass-fed beef, diced
- 1/2 cup barley
- 1 cup diced mushrooms
- 1 cup diced carrots
- 1 onion, diced
- 3 cloves garlic, minced
- 4 cups beef broth
- 1 tablespoon olive oil
- Salt and pepper to taste
- 1 teaspoon thyme

Allergens:
- None

DIRECTIONS

1. Rinse 1/2 cup of barley under cold water. Combine with 1 1/2 cups of water, bring to a boil, reduce heat, and simmer for 30 minutes until tender. Drain and set aside.
2. Dice the onion, carrots, mushrooms, and mince the garlic.
3. Heat olive oil in a pot over medium heat. Sauté onion, carrots, and mushrooms for 5-7 minutes until softened.
4. Add garlic and thyme, cook for another minute. Add beef broth, diced beef, and cooked barley. Bring to a boil, then simmer for 20 minutes. Season with salt and pepper. Serve hot.

Chicken and Quinoa Soup

Serves: 4 | Time: 45 min

Macronutrients (per serving):
Calories: 300
Protein: 20 g
Fat: 10 g
Carbs: 30 g

INGREDIENTS

- 1 cup cooked chicken breast, shredded
- 1/2 cup quinoa
- 1 cup diced tomatoes
- 1 cup spinach, chopped
- 1 onion, diced
- 3 cloves garlic, minced
- 4 cups chicken broth
- 1 tablespoon olive oil
- Salt and pepper to taste
- 1 teaspoon oregano

Allergens:
- None

DIRECTIONS

1. Rinse 1/2 cup of quinoa under cold water. Combine with 1 cup of water in a pot, bring to a boil, reduce heat, and simmer for 15 minutes until absorbed. Let it cool slightly.
2. Dice the onion and tomatoes, chop the spinach, and mince the garlic.
3. Heat olive oil in a large pot over medium heat. Sauté onion and tomatoes for 5-7 minutes until softened. Add garlic and oregano, cook for another minute.
4. Add chicken broth, shredded chicken, and quinoa. Bring to a boil, reduce heat, and simmer for 20 minutes. Stir in spinach, cook for 5 more minutes. Season with salt and pepper. Serve hot.

Meat Broths and Light Soups

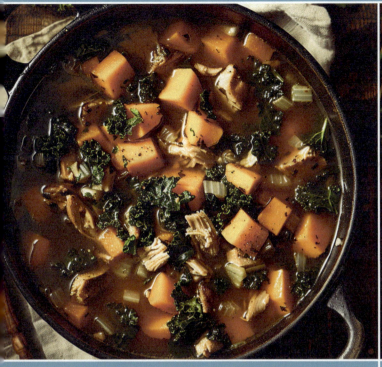
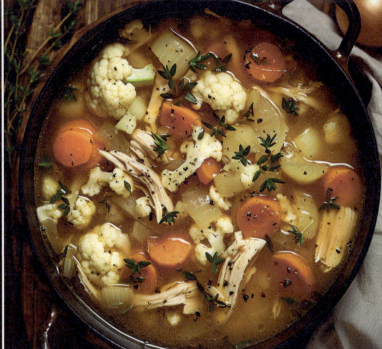

Turkey and Vegetable Broth

🍴 4   🕐 35 min   Macronutrients (per serving):   Protein: 18 g
Calories: 250   Fat: 8 g
Carbs: 25 g

INGREDIENTS

- 1 cup cooked turkey breast, shredded
- 2 cups kale, chopped
- 1 cup diced sweet potatoes
- 1 onion, diced
- 3 cloves garlic, minced
- 4 cups turkey broth
- 1 tablespoon olive oil
- Salt and pepper to taste
- 1 teaspoon turmeric

Allergens:
- None

DIRECTIONS

1. Dice the onion and sweet potatoes, chop the kale, and mince the garlic.
2. Heat olive oil in a large pot over medium heat. Add the onion and sweet potatoes, and sauté for 5-7 minutes until softened. Add the garlic and turmeric, and cook for another minute.
3. Add the turkey broth, shredded turkey, and chopped kale to the pot. Bring to a boil, then reduce the heat and simmer for 20 minutes. Season with salt and pepper to taste. Serve hot.

Chicken and Cauliflower Soup

🍴 4   🕐 30 min   Macronutrients (per serving):   Protein: 18 g
Calories: 240   Fat: 8 g
Carbs: 20 g

INGREDIENTS

- 1 cup cooked chicken breast, shredded
- 2 cups cauliflower florets
- 1 cup diced carrots
- 1 onion, diced
- 3 cloves garlic, minced
- 4 cups chicken broth
- 1 tablespoon olive oil
- Salt and pepper to taste
- 1 teaspoon thyme

Allergens:
- None

DIRECTIONS

1. Dice the onion and carrots, and mince the garlic.
2. Heat olive oil in a large pot over medium heat. Add the onion and carrots, and sauté for 5-7 minutes until softened. Add the garlic and thyme, and cook for another minute.
3. Add the chicken broth, shredded chicken, and cauliflower florets to the pot. Bring to a boil, then reduce the heat and simmer for 20 minutes. Season with salt and pepper to taste. Serve hot.

Seafood Soups

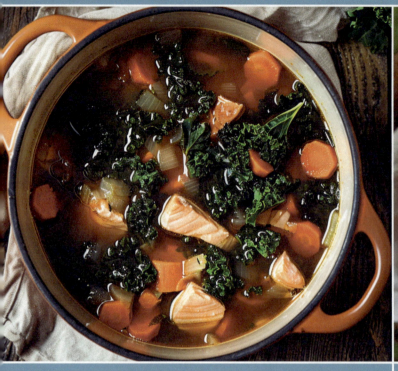

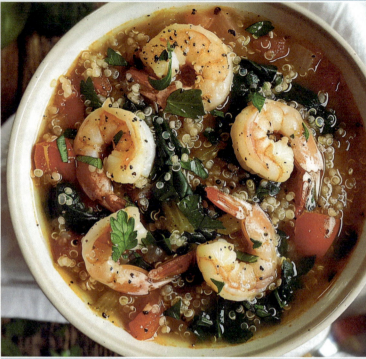

Salmon and Kale Soup

| 4 | 30 min | Macronutrients (per serving): Calories: 250 | Protein: 20 g Fat: 10 g Carbs: 15 g |

INGREDIENTS

- 1 cup cooked salmon, flaked
- 2 cups kale, chopped
- 1 cup diced carrots
- 1 onion, diced
- 3 cloves garlic, minced
- 4 cups vegetable broth
- 1 tablespoon olive oil
- 1 teaspoon turmeric
- Salt and pepper to taste

Allergens:
- Fish (salmon)

DIRECTIONS

1. Dice the onion and carrots, and mince the garlic.
2. Heat olive oil in a large pot over medium heat. Add the onion and carrots, and sauté for 5-7 minutes until softened. Add the garlic and turmeric, and cook for another minute.
3. Add the vegetable broth and bring to a boil. Reduce the heat and simmer for 15 minutes. Add the chopped kale and cook for another 5 minutes.
4. Stir in the flaked salmon and season with salt and pepper to taste.
5. Serve hot.

Shrimp and Quinoa Soup

| 4 | 40 min | Macronutrients (per serving): Calories: 300 | Protein: 20 g Fat: 8 g Carbs: 30 g |

INGREDIENTS

- 1 cup cooked shrimp, peeled and deveined
- 1/2 cup quinoa
- 1 cup diced tomatoes
- 1 cup spinach, chopped
- 1 onion, diced
- 3 cloves garlic, minced
- 4 cups vegetable broth
- 1 tablespoon olive oil
- Salt and pepper to taste
- 1 teaspoon ginger

Allergens:
- Shellfish (shrimp)

DIRECTIONS

1. Rinse 1/2 cup quinoa under cold water. Combine with 1 cup water in a pot, bring to a boil, reduce heat, and simmer for 15 minutes until absorbed. Let cool slightly.
2. Dice onion and tomatoes, chop spinach, and mince garlic.
3. Heat olive oil in a large pot over medium heat. Sauté onion and tomatoes for 5-7 minutes until softened. Add garlic and ginger, and cook for another minute.
4. Add vegetable broth, and bring to a boil. Reduce heat, and simmer for 15 minutes. Add spinach and quinoa, and cook for 5 more minutes.

Seafood Soups

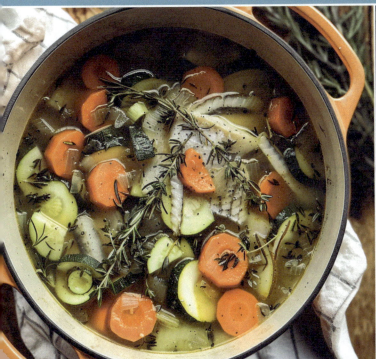

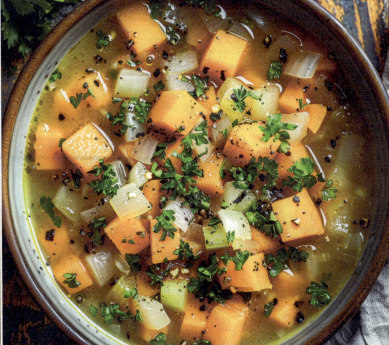

Mackerel and Vegetable Soup

4 | 30 min | Macronutrients (per serving): Calories: 270 | Protein: 22 g Fat: 12 g Carbs: 18 g

INGREDIENTS

- 1 cup cooked mackerel, flaked
- 1 cup diced zucchini
- 1 cup diced carrots
- 1 onion, diced
- 3 cloves garlic, minced
- 4 cups vegetable broth
- 1 tablespoon olive oil
- Salt and pepper to taste
- 1 teaspoon thyme

Allergens:
- Fish (mackerel)

DIRECTIONS

1. Dice the onion, carrots, and zucchini, and mince the garlic.
2. Heat olive oil in a large pot over medium heat. Add the onion, carrots, and zucchini, and sauté for 5-7 minutes until softened. Add the garlic and thyme, and cook for another minute.
3. Add the vegetable broth and bring to a boil. Reduce the heat and simmer for 20 minutes.
4. Stir in the flaked mackerel and season with salt and pepper to taste.
5. Serve hot.

Herring and Sweet Potato Soup

4 | 35 min | Macronutrients (per serving): Calories: 280 | Protein: 20 g Fat: 10 g Carbs: 30 g

INGREDIENTS

- 1 cup cooked herring, flaked
- 2 cups diced sweet potatoes
- 1 cup diced celery
- 1 onion, diced
- 3 cloves garlic, minced
- 4 cups vegetable broth
- 1 tablespoon olive oil
- Salt and pepper to taste
- 1 teaspoon turmeric

Allergens:
- Fish (herring)

DIRECTIONS

1. Dice the onion, sweet potatoes, and celery, and mince the garlic.
2. Heat olive oil in a large pot over medium heat. Add the onion, sweet potatoes, and celery, and sauté for 5-7 minutes until softened. Add the garlic and turmeric, and cook for another minute.
3. Add the vegetable broth and bring to a boil. Reduce the heat and simmer for 20 minutes until the sweet potatoes are tender.
4. Stir in the flaked herring and season with salt and pepper to taste. Serve hot.

Seafood Soups

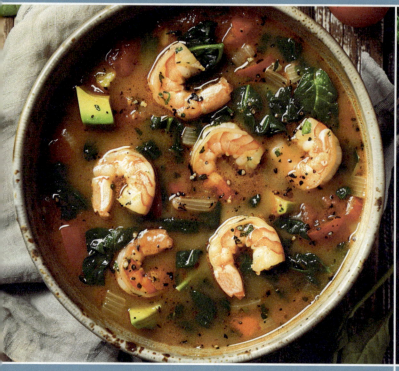

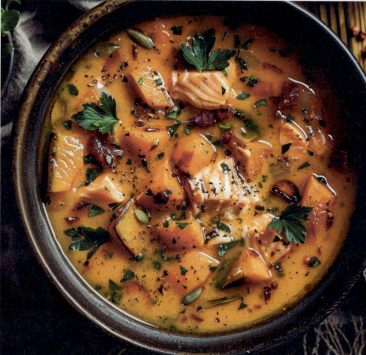

Shrimp and Avocado Soup

4 | 30 min | Macronutrients (per serving): Calories: 320 | Protein: 22 g Fat: 15 g Carbs: 28 g

INGREDIENTS
- 1 cup cooked shrimp
- 1 avocado, diced
- 1 cup diced tomatoes
- 1 cup spinach, chopped
- 1 onion, diced
- 3 cloves garlic, minced
- 4 cups vegetable broth
- 1 tablespoon olive oil
- Salt and pepper to taste
- 1 teaspoon ginger

Allergens:
- Shellfish (shrimp)

DIRECTIONS
1. Dice the onion and tomatoes, chop the spinach, and mince the garlic.
2. Heat olive oil in a large pot over medium heat. Add the onion and tomatoes, and sauté for 5-7 minutes until softened. Add the garlic and ginger, and cook for another minute.
3. Add the vegetable broth and bring to a boil. Reduce the heat and simmer for 15 minutes.
4. Stir in the cooked shrimp, diced avocado, and chopped spinach. Cook for another 5 minutes. Season with salt and pepper to taste.
5. Serve hot.

Salmon and Pumpkin Soup

4 | 35 min | Macronutrients (per serving): Calories: 300 | Protein: 20 g Fat: 12 g Carbs: 28 g

INGREDIENTS
- 1 cup cooked salmon, flaked
- 2 cups diced pumpkin
- 1 cup diced red bell pepper
- 1 onion, diced
- 3 cloves garlic, minced
- 4 cups vegetable broth
- 1 tablespoon olive oil
- Salt and pepper to taste
- 1 teaspoon turmeric

Allergens:
- Fish (salmon)

DIRECTIONS
1. Dice the onion, pumpkin, and red bell pepper, and mince the garlic.
2. Heat olive oil in a large pot over medium heat. Add the onion, pumpkin, and red bell pepper, and sauté for 5-7 minutes until softened. Add the garlic and turmeric, and cook for another minute.
3. Add the vegetable broth and bring to a boil. Reduce the heat and simmer for 20 minutes until the pumpkin is tender.
4. Stir in the flaked salmon and season with salt and pepper to taste.
5. Serve hot.

Cream Soups

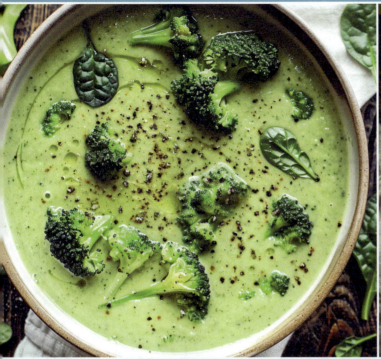

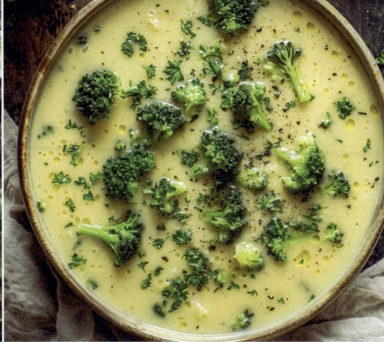

Creamy Broccoli and Spinach Soup

Serves: 4 | Time: 30 min | Macronutrients (per serving): Calories: 150 | Protein: 5 g | Fat: 7 g | Carbs: 18 g

INGREDIENTS

- 2 cups broccoli florets
- 2 cups spinach, chopped
- 1 onion, diced
- 3 cloves garlic, minced
- 4 cups vegetable broth
- 1 cup unsweetened almond milk
- 1 tablespoon olive oil
- 1 teaspoon turmeric
- Salt and pepper to taste

Allergens:
- Nuts (almond milk)

DIRECTIONS

1. Dice the onion and mince the garlic.
2. Heat olive oil in a large pot over medium heat. Add the onion and sauté for 5-7 minutes until softened. Add the garlic and cook for another minute.
3. Add the broccoli florets and vegetable broth. Bring to a boil, then reduce the heat and simmer for 15 minutes until the broccoli is tender.
4. Add the chopped spinach and almond milk. Use an immersion blender to puree the soup until smooth. Season with salt, pepper, and turmeric.
5. Serve hot.

Creamy Cauliflower and Garlic Soup

Serves: 4 | Time: 35 min | Macronutrients (per serving): Calories: 170 | Protein: 4 g | Fat: 10 g | Carbs: 20 g

INGREDIENTS

- 1 large cauliflower, chopped
- 1 onion, diced
- 4 cloves garlic, minced
- 4 cups vegetable broth
- 1 cup unsweetened coconut milk
- 1 tablespoon olive oil
- 1 teaspoon thyme
- Salt and pepper to taste

Allergens:
- None

DIRECTIONS

1. Dice the onion and mince the garlic.
2. Heat olive oil in a large pot over medium heat. Add the onion and garlic, and sauté for 5-7 minutes until softened.
3. Add the chopped cauliflower and vegetable broth. Bring to a boil, then reduce the heat and simmer for 20 minutes until the cauliflower is tender.
4. Add the coconut milk and thyme. Use an immersion blender to puree the soup until smooth. Season with salt and pepper. Serve hot.

Cream Soups

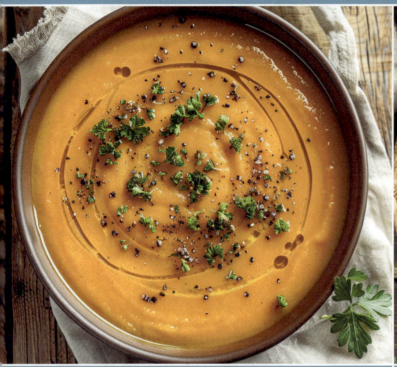

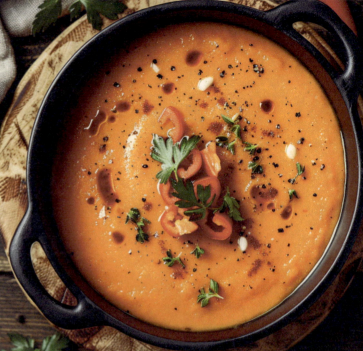

Creamy Pumpkin and Carrot Soup

| 4 | 35 min | Macronutrients (per serving): Calories: 180 | Protein: 4 g Fat: 7 g Carbs: 28 g |

INGREDIENTS

- 2 cups pumpkin, diced
- 2 cups carrots, sliced
- 1 onion, diced
- 3 cloves garlic, minced
- 4 cups vegetable broth
- 1 cup unsweetened oat milk
- 1 tablespoon olive oil
- 1 teaspoon ginger, grated
- Salt and pepper to taste

Allergens:
- None

DIRECTIONS

1. Dice the onion and garlic, and grate the ginger.
2. Heat olive oil in a large pot over medium heat. Add the onion, garlic, and ginger, and sauté for 5-7 minutes until softened.
3. Add the pumpkin, carrots, and vegetable broth. Bring to a boil, then reduce the heat and simmer for 20 minutes until the vegetables are tender.
4. Add the oat milk. Use an immersion blender to puree the soup until smooth. Season with salt and pepper. Serve hot.

Creamy Sweet Potato and Red Pepper Soup

| 4 | 35 min | Macronutrients (per serving): Calories: 190 | Protein: 3 g Fat: 8 g Carbs: 29 g |

INGREDIENTS

- 2 large sweet potatoes, peeled and diced
- 1 red bell pepper, diced
- 1 onion, diced
- 3 cloves garlic, minced
- 4 cups vegetable broth
- 1 tablespoon olive oil
- 1 teaspoon turmeric
- 1 cup unsweetened coconut milk
- Salt and pepper to taste

Allergens:
- None

DIRECTIONS

1. Dice the onion, red bell pepper, and garlic.
2. Heat olive oil in a large pot over medium heat. Add the onion, red bell pepper, and garlic, and sauté for 5-7 minutes until softened.
3. Add the sweet potatoes and vegetable broth. Bring to a boil, then reduce the heat and simmer for 20 minute s until the sweet potatoes are tender.
4. Add the coconut milk and turmeric. Use an immersion blender to puree the soup until smooth. Season with salt and pepper. Serve hot.

Cream Soups

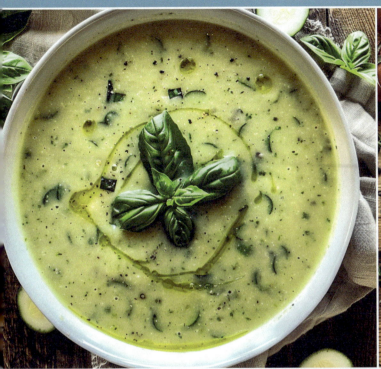

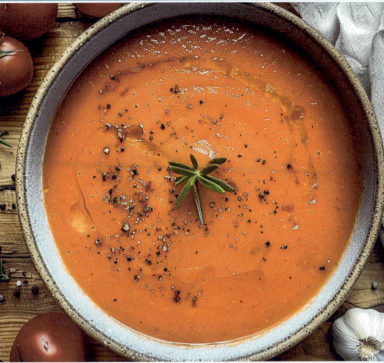

Creamy Zucchini and Basil Soup

🍴 4 | 🕒 30 min | Macronutrients (per serving): Calories: 140 | Protein: 4 g / Fat: 6 g / Carbs: 18 g

INGREDIENTS

- 4 cups zucchini, sliced
- 1 onion, diced
- 3 cloves garlic, minced
- 4 cups vegetable broth
- 1 cup unsweetened almond milk
- 1/4 cup fresh basil, chopped
- 1 tablespoon olive oil
- Salt and pepper to taste

Allergens:
- Nuts (almond milk)

DIRECTIONS

1. Dice the onion and garlic, and chop the basil.
2. Heat olive oil in a large pot over medium heat. Add the onion and garlic, and sauté for 5-7 minutes until softened.
3. Add the zucchini and vegetable broth. Bring to a boil, then reduce the heat and simmer for 15 minutes until the zucchini is tender.
4. Add the almond milk and fresh basil. Use an immersion blender to puree the soup until smooth. Season with salt and pepper. Serve hot.

Creamy Tomato and Red Pepper Soup

🍴 4 | 🕒 35 min | Macronutrients (per serving): Calories: 160 | Protein: 4 g / Fat: 7 g / Carbs: 22 g

INGREDIENTS

- 4 cups tomatoes, diced
- 2 red bell peppers, diced
- 1 onion, diced
- 3 cloves garlic, minced
- 4 cups vegetable broth
- 1 cup unsweetened oat milk
- 1 tablespoon olive oil
- 1 teaspoon thyme
- Salt and pepper to taste

Allergens:
- None

DIRECTIONS

1. Dice the onion, tomatoes, red bell peppers, and garlic.
2. Heat olive oil in a large pot over medium heat. Add the onion, garlic, tomatoes, and red bell peppers, and sauté for 5-7 minutes until softened.
3. Add the vegetable broth and bring to a boil. Reduce the heat and simmer for 20 minutes until the vegetables are tender.
4. Add the oat milk and thyme. Use an immersion blender to puree the soup until smooth. Season with salt and pepper. Serve hot.

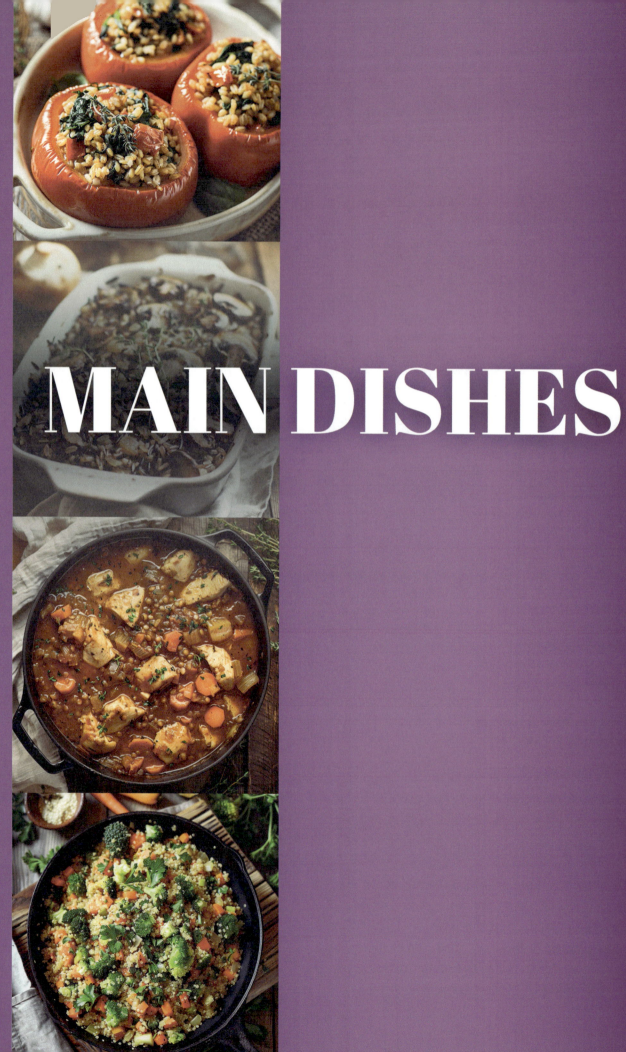

MAIN DISHES

Fish and Seafood Dishes

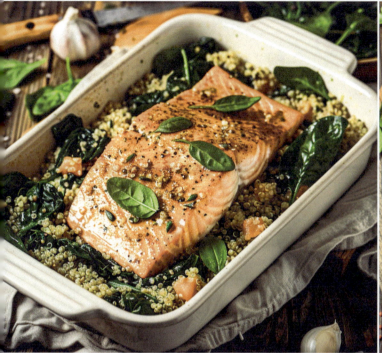

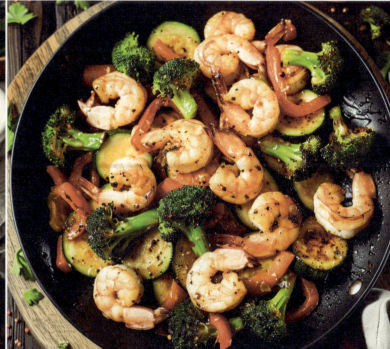

Baked Salmon with Quinoa and Spinach

| 2 | 35 min | Macronutrients (per serving):
Calories: 450 | Protein: 35 g
Fat: 18 g
Carbs: 40 g |

INGREDIENTS

- 2 salmon fillets
- 1 cup quinoa
- 2 cups spinach, chopped
- 1 onion, diced
- 2 cloves garlic, minced
- 1 tablespoon olive oil
- Salt and pepper to taste
- 1 teaspoon turmeric

Allergens:
- Fish (salmon)

DIRECTIONS

1. Rinse 1 cup of quinoa under cold water. Combine with 2 cups of water, bring to a boil, then simmer for 15 minutes until absorbed. Cool slightly.
2. Preheat oven to 375°F (190°C). Place salmon on a baking sheet, drizzle with olive oil, season with salt, pepper, and turmeric. Bake for 15-20 minutes until cooked.
3. Heat olive oil in a pan over medium heat. Sauté diced onion and minced garlic for 5-7 minutes until softened. Add chopped spinach and cook for 2-3 minutes until wilted.
4. Serve the salmon on quinoa and sautéed spinach.

Shrimp and Vegetable Stir-Fry

| 4 | 20 min | Macronutrients (per serving):
Calories: 300 | Protein: 30 g
Fat: 10 g
Carbs: 20 g |

INGREDIENTS

- 1 lb shrimp, peeled and deveined
- 1 cup broccoli florets
- 1 red bell pepper, sliced
- 1 zucchini, sliced
- 2 cloves garlic, minced
- 1 tablespoon olive oil
- 1 teaspoon ginger, grated
- Salt and pepper to taste

Allergens:
- Shellfish (shrimp)

DIRECTIONS

1. Mince the garlic and grate the ginger.
2. Heat olive oil in a large pan over medium heat. Add the shrimp and cook for 3-4 minutes until pink and opaque. Remove from the pan and set aside.
3. In the same pan, add more olive oil if needed, and sauté the garlic and ginger for 1 minute. Add broccoli, red bell pepper, and zucchini, and cook for 5-7 minutes until tender.
4. Return the shrimp to the pan, mix well, and season with salt and pepper. Serve immediately.

Fish and Seafood Dishes

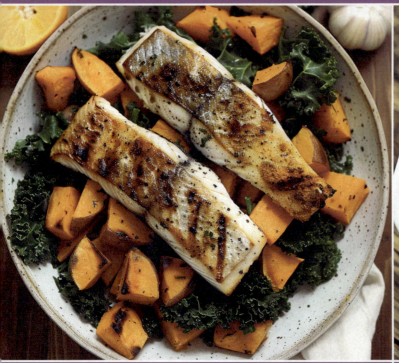

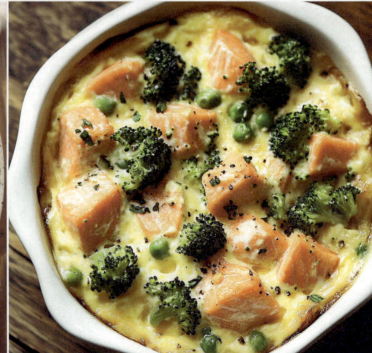

Mackerel with Sweet Potato and Kale

🍴 2   ⏱ 35 min   Macronutrients (per serving):   Protein: 30 g   Fat: 18 g   Calories: 400   Carbs: 30 g

INGREDIENTS

- 2 mackerel fillets
- 2 cups sweet potatoes, diced
- 2 cups kale, chopped
- 1 onion, diced
- 2 cloves garlic, minced
- 1 tablespoon olive oil
- 1 teaspoon turmeric
- Salt and pepper to taste

Allergens:
- Fish (mackerel)

DIRECTIONS

1. Preheat oven to 400°F (200°C). Toss diced sweet potatoes with olive oil, salt, and turmeric. Roast on a baking sheet for 25-30 minutes until tender.
2. Season mackerel fillets with salt and pepper. Heat olive oil in a pan over medium heat, cook mackerel for 3-4 minutes per side until done. Set aside.
3. In the same pan, sauté diced onion and minced garlic for 5-7 minutes until softened. Add chopped kale and cook for 2-3 minutes until wilted.
4. Serve mackerel with roasted sweet potatoes and sautéed kale.

Egg-Based Salmon Casserole

🍴 3   ⏱ 40 min   Macronutrients (per serving):   Protein: 25 g   Fat: 18 g   Calories: 280   Carbs: 4 g

INGREDIENTS

- 1 lb fresh salmon fillet, cubed
- 4 large eggs
- 1/2 cup broccoli florets, chopped
- 1/2 small onion, finely chopped
- 1 clove garlic, minced
- 1/4 cup Greek yogurt (unsweetened)
- 1 tbsp olive oil
- 1/2 tsp salt
- 1/2 tsp black pepper

Allergens:
- Fish (Salmon)
- Eggs
- Dairy (Greek Yogurt)

DIRECTIONS

1. Preheat your oven to 375°F (190°C).
2. Heat olive oil in a skillet over medium heat. Add onions and garlic, sauté until softened. Add broccoli and cook for 3-4 minutes until slightly tender.
3. In a mixing bowl, beat the eggs and stir in Greek yogurt, salt, and pepper.
4. In the same bowl, add the sautéed vegetables and salmon cubes. Stir until everything is evenly coated with the egg mixture.
5. Pour the mixture into a greased baking dish and spread it out evenly. Bake for 25-30 minutes, or until the eggs are set and the top is golden brown.
6. Let the casserole cool slightly before serving.

Lean Meat Dishes

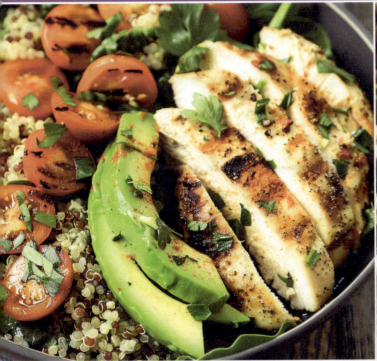

Grilled Chicken with Quinoa and Avocado

🍴 2	⏰ 30 min	Macronutrients (per serving): Calories: 450	Protein: 40 g Fat: 20 g Carbs: 35 g

INGREDIENTS

- 2 chicken breasts
- 1 cup quinoa
- 1 avocado, diced
- 1 cup cherry tomatoes, halved
- 1 cup spinach, chopped
- 1 tablespoon olive oil
- 1 teaspoon turmeric
- Salt and pepper to taste

Allergens:
- None

DIRECTIONS

1. Rinse 1 cup of quinoa under cold water. Combine with 2 cups of water in a pot, bring to a boil, then reduce heat and simmer for 15 minutes until water is absorbed. Let it cool slightly.
2. Preheat the grill to medium-high heat. Season the chicken breasts with olive oil, salt, pepper, and turmeric. Grill for 6-7 minutes on each side or until fully cooked.
3. In a large bowl, combine cooked quinoa, diced avocado, halved cherry tomatoes, and chopped spinach.
4. Slice the grilled chicken and serve over the quinoa salad. Drizzle with additional olive oil if desired.

Baked Turkey Meatballs with Sweet Potato

🍴 4	⏰ 40 min	Macronutrients (per serving): Calories: 400	Protein: 35 g Fat: 15 g Carbs: 30 g

INGREDIENTS

- 1 lb ground turkey
- 1 egg, beaten
- 1/2 cup whole grain flour
- 1 onion, diced
- 2 cloves garlic, minced
- 2 cups sweet potatoes, diced
- 1 teaspoon turmeric
- 1 tablespoon olive oil
- Salt and pepper to taste

Allergens:
- Eggs
- Whole grain flour

DIRECTIONS

1. Preheat the oven to 375°F (190°C). In a large bowl, combine ground turkey, beaten egg, diced onion, minced garlic, whole grain flour, salt, pepper, and turmeric. Mix well and form into meatballs.
2. Place the meatballs on a baking sheet lined with parchment paper. Bake for 20-25 minutes until fully cooked.
3. While the meatballs are baking, toss the diced sweet potatoes with olive oil, salt, and pepper. Spread on a separate baking sheet and roast for 25-30 minutes until tender.
4. Serve the baked turkey meatballs with roasted sweet potatoes.

Lean Meat Dishes

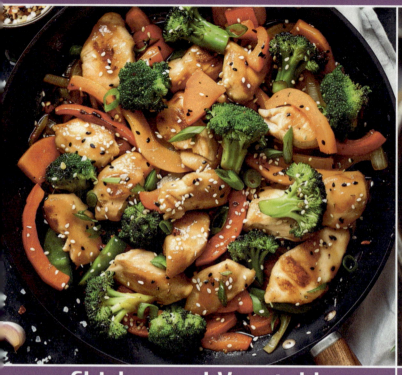

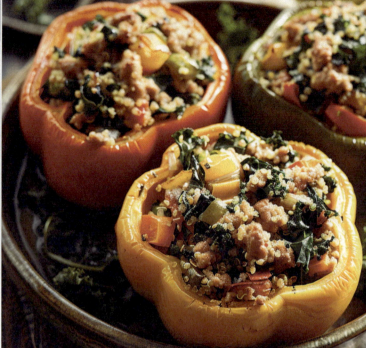

Chicken and Vegetable Stir-Fry

4 | 20 min | Macronutrients (per serving): Calories: 350 | Protein: 30 g Fat: 15 g Carbs: 20 g

INGREDIENTS

- 2 chicken breasts, sliced
- 1 red bell pepper, sliced
- 1 cup broccoli florets
- 1 cup carrots, julienned
- 1 onion, sliced
- 2 cloves garlic, minced
- 1 tablespoon olive oil
- 1 teaspoon ginger
- Salt and pepper to taste

Allergens:
- None

DIRECTIONS

1. Slice chicken breasts, bell pepper, broccoli, carrots, and onion. Mince garlic and grate ginger.
2. Heat olive oil in a large pan over medium heat. Add chicken and cook for 5-7 minutes until no longer pink. Remove and set aside.
3. In the same pan, add more olive oil if needed, and sauté garlic and ginger for 1 minute. Add bell pepper, broccoli, carrots, and onion, and cook for 5-7 minutes until tender.
4. Return chicken to the pan, mix well, and season with salt and pepper. Serve immediately.

Turkey and Kale Stuffed Peppers

4 | 40 min | Macronutrients (per serving): Calories: 400 | Protein: 30 g Fat: 15 g Carbs: 35 g

INGREDIENTS

- 1 lb ground turkey
- 4 large bell peppers
- 1 cup cooked quinoa
- 2 cups kale, chopped
- 1 onion, diced
- 2 cloves garlic, minced
- 1 tablespoon olive oil
- 1 teaspoon turmeric
- Salt and pepper to taste

Allergens:
- None

DIRECTIONS

1. Preheat the oven to 375°F (190°C). Cut the tops off the bell peppers and remove the seeds.
2. Heat olive oil in a pan over medium heat. Sauté diced onion and minced garlic for 5-7 minutes until softened. Add ground turkey and cook until browned. Stir in chopped kale, cooked quinoa, salt, pepper, and turmeric.
3. Fill bell peppers with the mixture, place in a baking dish, and cover with foil.
4. Bake for 25-30 minutes until tender. Serve hot.

Lean Meat Dishes

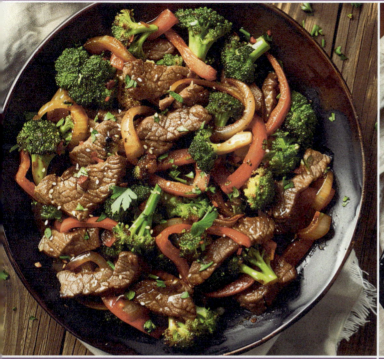

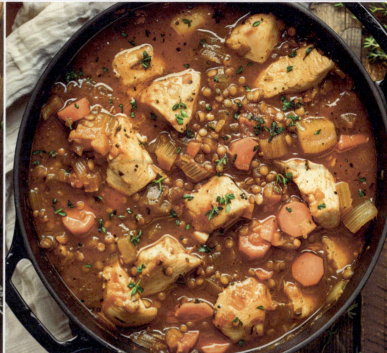

Beef and Broccoli Stir-Fry

Serves: 4 | Time: 20 min

Macronutrients (per serving):
Calories: 350
Protein: 25 g
Fat: 18 g
Carbs: 20 g

INGREDIENTS

- 1 lb grass-fed beef, thinly sliced
- 2 cups broccoli florets
- 1 red bell pepper, sliced
- 1 onion, sliced
- 2 cloves garlic, minced
- 1 tablespoon olive oil
- 1 tablespoon soy sauce (optional for flavor)
- Salt and pepper to taste

Allergens:
- None

DIRECTIONS

1. Thinly slice the beef, broccoli, red bell pepper, and onion. Mince the garlic.
2. Heat olive oil in a large pan over medium-high heat. Add the sliced beef and cook for 3-4 minutes until browned. Remove from the pan and set aside.
3. In the same pan, add more olive oil if needed, and sauté the garlic for 1 minute. Add the broccoli, red bell pepper, and onion, and cook for 5-7 minutes until tender.
4. Return the beef to the pan, mix well, and season with soy sauce, salt, and pepper. Serve immediately.

Chicken and Lentil Stew

Serves: 4 | Time: 40 min

Macronutrients (per serving):
Calories: 400
Protein: 35 g
Fat: 10 g
Carbs: 40 g

INGREDIENTS

- 2 chicken breasts, diced
- 1 cup lentils, rinsed and drained
- 2 carrots, sliced
- 2 celery stalks, sliced
- 1 onion, diced
- 3 cloves garlic, minced
- 4 cups chicken broth
- 1 tablespoon olive oil
- 1 teaspoon turmeric
- Salt and pepper to taste

Allergens:
- None

DIRECTIONS

1. Dice the chicken, slice the carrots and celery, and mince the garlic.
2. Heat olive oil in a large pot over medium heat. Add the diced chicken and cook for 5-7 minutes until browned.
3. Add the diced onion, garlic, carrots, and celery to the pot. Cook for another 5 minutes until the vegetables are softened. Add the lentils, chicken broth, turmeric, salt, and pepper. Bring to a boil, then reduce the heat and simmer for 30 minutes until the lentils are tender. Serve hot.

Vegetarian Dishes

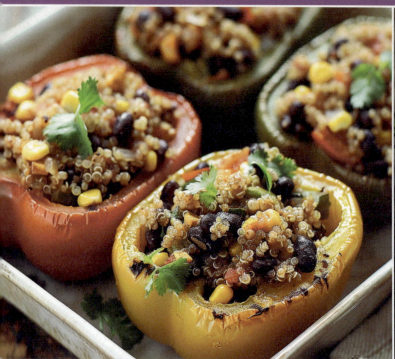
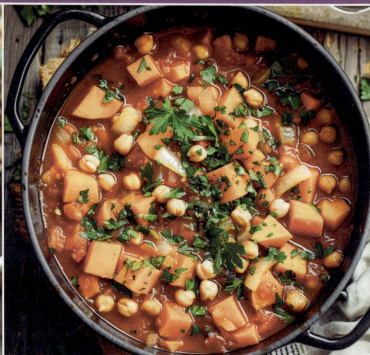

Stuffed Bell Peppers with Black Beans and Corn

4 | 130 min | Macronutrients (per serving): Calories: 350 | Protein: 12 g | Fat: 10 g | Carbs: 55 g

INGREDIENTS
- 4 bell peppers (any color), tops cut off and seeds removed
- 1 cup black beans, cooked
- 1 cup corn kernels
- 1 cup quinoa, cooked
- 1 onion, diced
- 2 cloves garlic, minced
- 1 tablespoon olive oil
- 1 teaspoon cumin
- Salt and pepper to taste

Allergens:
- None

DIRECTIONS
1. Rinse 1 cup of quinoa and cook with 2 cups of water for 15 minutes, then cool slightly.
2. Soak 1 cup dried black beans overnight, then drain, rinse, and cook for 60-90 minutes, or rinse and drain canned beans.
3. Preheat oven to 375°F (190°C).
4. Sauté diced onion and minced garlic in olive oil for 5-7 minutes. Add black beans, corn, quinoa, cumin, salt, and pepper, and mix well.
5. Fill bell peppers with the mixture, place in a baking dish, cover with foil, and bake for 25-30 minutes until tender. Serve hot.

Chickpea and Sweet Potato Stew

4 | 45 min | Macronutrients (per serving): Calories: 400 | Protein: 10 g | Fat: 10 g | Carbs: 70 g

INGREDIENTS
- 1 can chickpeas (15 oz), rinsed and drained
- 2 cups sweet potatoes, diced
- 1 onion, diced
- 2 cloves garlic, minced
- 2 cups vegetable broth
- 1 can diced tomatoes (15 oz)
- 1 tablespoon olive oil
- 1 teaspoon turmeric
- 1 teaspoon cumin
- Salt and pepper to taste

Allergens:
- None

DIRECTIONS
1. Heat olive oil in a large pot over medium heat. Add the diced onion and minced garlic, and sauté for 5-7 minutes until softened.
2. Add the diced sweet potatoes, turmeric, cumin, and vegetable broth to the pot. Bring to a boil, then reduce heat and simmer for 20-25 minutes until the sweet potatoes are tender.
3. Stir in the chickpeas (canned, rinsed, and drained) and diced tomatoes. Cook for another 10 minutes. Season with salt and pepper to taste.
4. Serve hot.

Vegetarian Dishes

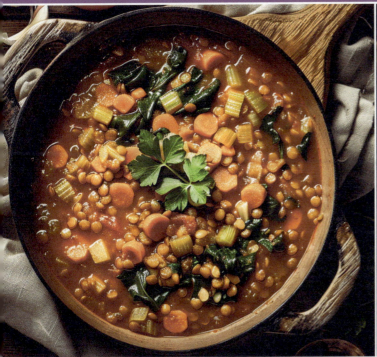

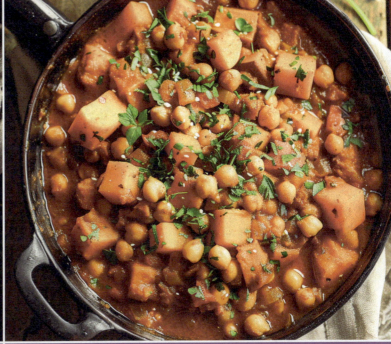

Lentil and Vegetable Stew

🍴 4 ⏱ 40 min Macronutrients (per serving): Calories: 300 Protein: 15 g Fat: 6 g Carbs: 50 g

INGREDIENTS

- 1 cup lentils, rinsed and drained
- 1 cup carrots, diced
- 1 cup celery, diced
- 1 onion, diced
- 2 cloves garlic, minced
- 2 cups spinach, chopped
- 4 cups vegetable broth
- 1 tablespoon olive oil
- 1 teaspoon turmeric
- Salt and pepper to taste

Allergens:
- None

DIRECTIONS

1. Heat olive oil in a large pot over medium heat. Add the diced onion, celery, and carrots, and sauté for 5-7 minutes until softened. Add the minced garlic and cook for another minute.
2. Add the lentils, turmeric, and vegetable broth to the pot. Bring to a boil, then reduce heat and simmer for 20-25 minutes until the lentils are tender.
3. Stir in the chopped spinach and cook for another 5 minutes until wilted. Season with salt and pepper to taste. Serve hot.

Chickpea and Sweet Potato Curry

🍴 4 ⏱ 45 min Macronutrients (per serving): Calories: 400 Protein: 10 g Fat: 10 g Carbs: 70 g

INGREDIENTS

- 1 can chickpeas (15 oz), rinsed and drained
- 2 cups sweet potatoes
- 1 onion, diced
- 2 cloves garlic, minced
- 1 can diced tomatoes (15 oz)
- 1 can coconut milk (400 ml)
- 2 cups vegetable broth
- 1 tablespoon olive oil
- 1 teaspoon turmeric
- 1 teaspoon cumin
- 1 teaspoon ginger, grated
- Salt and pepper to taste

Allergens:
- None

DIRECTIONS

1. Heat olive oil in a large pot over medium heat. Add the diced onion and minced garlic, and sauté for 5-7 minutes until softened. Add the grated ginger and cook for another minute.
2. Add the diced sweet potatoes, turmeric, cumin, and vegetable broth to the pot. Bring to a boil, then reduce heat and simmer for 20 minutes until the sweet potatoes are tender.
3. Stir in the chickpeas, diced tomatoes, and coconut milk. Cook for another 10 minutes. Season with salt and pepper to taste. Serve hot.

Vegetarian Dishes

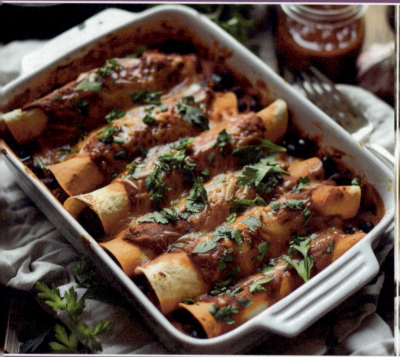

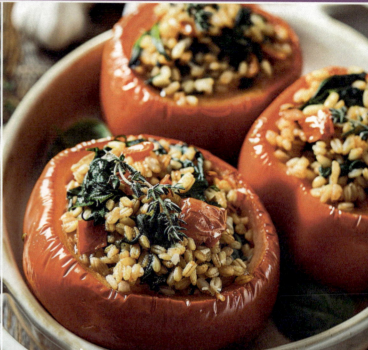

Black Bean and Sweet Potato Enchiladas (with Tomato Sauce)

 4   45 min

Macronutrients (per serving):
Calories: 400
Protein: 12 g
Fat: 12 g
Carbs: 60 g

INGREDIENTS

- 1 can black beans (15 oz), rinsed and drained
- 2 cups sweet potatoes, diced
- 1 onion, diced
- 2 cloves garlic, minced
- 1 red bell pepper, diced
- 1 cup tomato sauce
- 8 whole grain tortillas
- 1 tablespoon olive oil
- 1 teaspoon cumin
- 1 teaspoon chili powder
- Salt and pepper to taste

Allergens:
- Whole grain tortillas

DIRECTIONS

1. Heat olive oil in a large pan over medium heat. Add diced onion, minced garlic, and diced red bell pepper, and sauté for 5-7 minutes until softened.
2. Add diced sweet potatoes and cook for another 10 minutes until tender. Add black beans, cumin, chili powder, salt, and pepper. Cook for 5 minutes until heated through.
3. Preheat oven to 375°F (190°C). Fill each tortilla with the mixture, roll up, and place in a baking dish. Pour tomato sauce over the top.
4. Cover with foil and bake for 20-25 minutes until heated through. Serve hot.

Barley and Spinach Stuffed Peppers

4   70 min

Macronutrients (per serving):
Calories: 300
Protein: 8 g
Fat: 10 g
Carbs: 45 g

INGREDIENTS

- 4 bell peppers (any color), tops cut off and seeds removed
- 1 cup barley
- 2 cups spinach, chopped
- 1 onion, diced
- 2 cloves garlic, minced
- 2 cups vegetable broth
- 1 tablespoon olive oil
- 1 teaspoon thyme
- Salt and pepper to taste

Allergens:
- None

DIRECTIONS

1. Combine 1 cup of barley with 2 cups of vegetable broth, bring to a boil, reduce heat, and simmer for 45 minutes until tender and liquid is absorbed.
2. Heat olive oil in a large pan over medium heat, sauté diced onion and minced garlic for 5-7 minutes until softened. Add chopped spinach and thyme, cooking until wilted, about 5 minutes.
3. Preheat oven to 375°F (190°C). Mix cooked barley with spinach mixture, fill each bell pepper, place in a baking dish, cover with foil, and bake for 25-30 minutes until tender. Serve hot.

Vegetarian Dishes

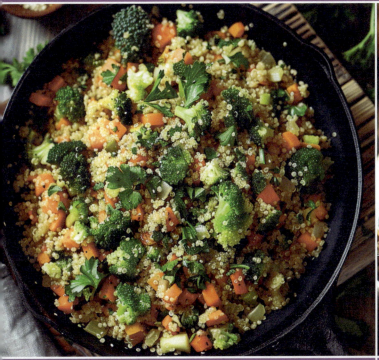

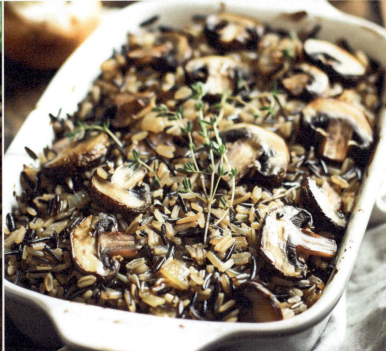

Quinoa and Vegetable Pilaf

🍴 4 | 🕐 30 min | Macronutrients (per serving): Calories: 350 | Protein: 10 g, Fat: 10 g, Carbs: 55 g

INGREDIENTS

- 1 cup quinoa
- 1 cup broccoli florets
- 1 cup carrots, diced
- 1 cup bell peppers (red, yellow, green), diced
- 1 onion, diced
- 2 cloves garlic, minced
- 1 tablespoon olive oil
- 1 teaspoon turmeric
- Salt and pepper to taste

Allergens:
- None

DIRECTIONS

1. Rinse 1 cup of quinoa under cold water. Combine with 2 cups of water in a pot, bring to a boil, then reduce heat and simmer for 15 minutes until water is absorbed. Let it cool slightly.
2. Heat olive oil in a large pan over medium heat. Add the diced onion and minced garlic, and sauté for 5-7 minutes until softened. Add the carrots and bell peppers, and cook for another 5 minutes until tender.
3. Add the cooked quinoa and broccoli florets to the pan. Season with turmeric, salt, and pepper. Cook for another 5 minutes until the broccoli is tender.
4. Serve hot.

Wild Rice and Mushroom Casserole

🍴 4 | 🕐 70 min | Macronutrients (per serving): Calories: 300 | Protein: 8 g, Fat: 10 g, Carbs: 45 g

INGREDIENTS

- 1 cup wild rice
- 2 cups mushrooms, sliced
- 1 onion, diced
- 2 cloves garlic, minced
- 2 cups vegetable broth
- 1 tablespoon olive oil
- 1 teaspoon thyme
- Salt and pepper to taste

Allergens:
- None

DIRECTIONS

1. Combine 1 cup of wild rice with 2 cups of vegetable broth in a pot, bring to a boil, reduce heat, and simmer for 45 minutes until tender and liquid is absorbed.
2. Heat olive oil in a large pan over medium heat, add diced onion and minced garlic, and sauté for 5-7 minutes until softened. Add sliced mushrooms and thyme, and cook for another 10 minutes until tender.
3. Preheat the oven to 375°F (190°C). Combine cooked wild rice and sautéed vegetables in a baking dish, season with salt and pepper, and bake for 20 minutes until heated through. Serve hot.

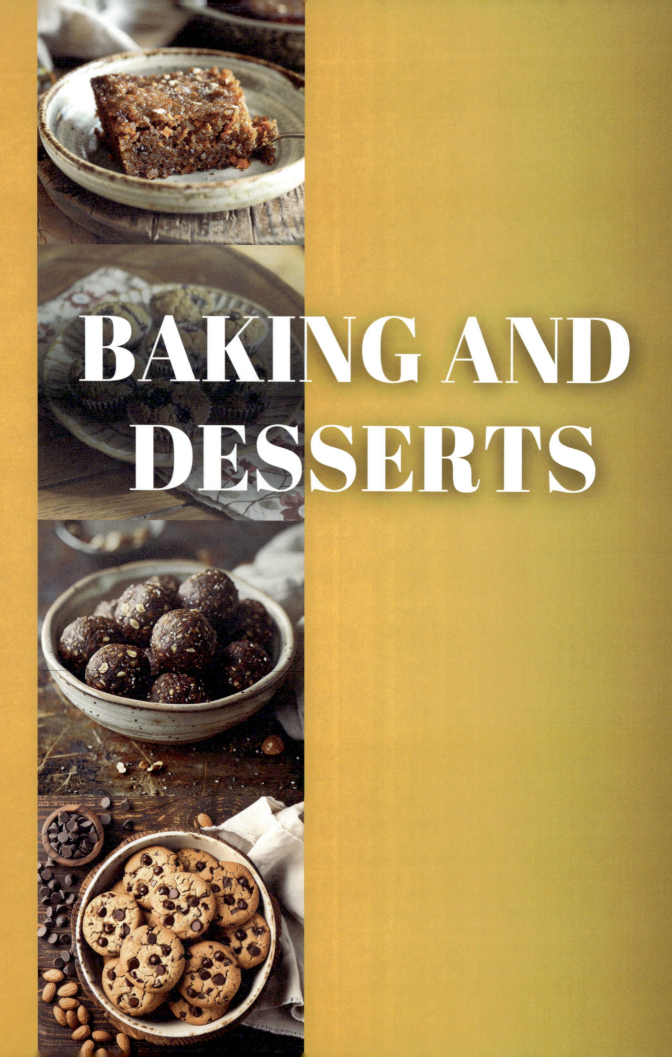

BAKING AND DESSERTS

Gluten-Free Baking

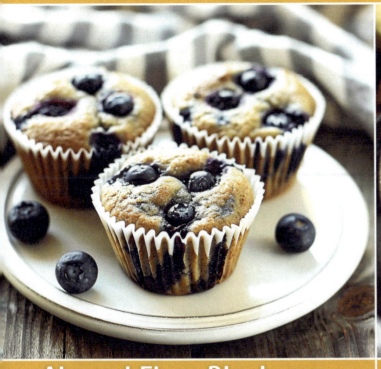

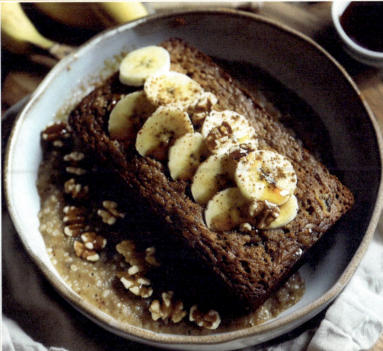

Almond Flour Blueberry Muffins

12 muffins | 30 min | Macronutrients (per serving): Calories: 200 | Protein: 6 g, Fat: 14 g, Carbs: 15 g

INGREDIENTS

- 2 cups almond flour
- 2 large eggs
- 1/4 cup honey or maple syrup
- 1/4 cup unsweetened almond milk
- 1 teaspoon vanilla extract
- 1/2 teaspoon baking soda
- 1 cup fresh blueberries

Allergens:
- Eggs
- Nuts (almond flour, almond milk)

DIRECTIONS

1. Preheat the oven to 350°F (175°C) and line a muffin tin with paper liners.
2. In a large bowl, whisk together eggs, honey or maple syrup, almond milk, and vanilla extract.
3. In another bowl, mix almond flour and baking soda.
4. Add the dry ingredients to the wet ingredients and mix until just combined. Fold in the blueberries.
5. Fill the muffin cups about 3/4 full with the batter. Bake for 20-25 minutes, or until a toothpick inserted into the center comes out clean.
6. Let the muffins cool in the tin for 10 minutes before transferring to a wire rack to cool completely.

Buckwheat Banana Bread

10 slices | 60 min | Macronutrients (per serving): Calories: 220 | Protein: 5 g, Fat: 10 g, Carbs: 30 g

INGREDIENTS

- 2 cups buckwheat flour
- 3 ripe bananas, mashed
- 2 large eggs
- 1/4 cup honey or maple syrup
- 1/4 cup coconut oil, melted
- 1 teaspoon vanilla extract
- 1 teaspoon baking soda
- 1/2 teaspoon cinnamon

Allergens:
- Eggs

DIRECTIONS

1. Preheat the oven to 350°F (175°C) and grease a loaf pan. In a large bowl, combine mashed bananas, eggs, honey or maple syrup, melted coconut oil, and vanilla extract.
2. In another bowl, mix buckwheat flour, baking soda, and cinnamon.
3. Add the dry ingredients to the wet ingredients and mix until just combined.
4. Pour the batter into the prepared loaf pan and bake for 45-50 minutes, or until a toothpick inserted into the center comes out clean.
5. Let cool in the pan for 10 minutes, then transfer to a wire rack to cool completely.

Gluten-Free Baking

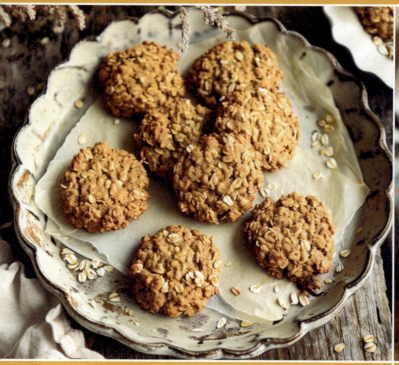

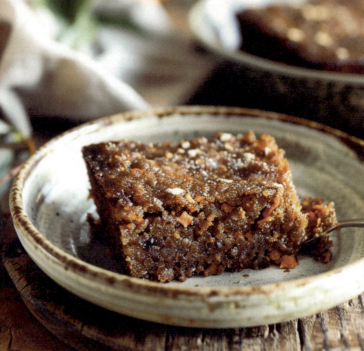

Pumpkin and Oat Cookies

20 cookies | 20 min | Macronutrients (per serving): Calories: 100 | Protein: 2 g Fat: 5 g Carbs: 12 g

INGREDIENTS

- 1 cup pumpkin puree
- 1 cup oats
- 1/4 cup honey or maple syrup
- 1/4 cup coconut oil, melted
- 1 teaspoon cinnamon
- 1/2 teaspoon ginger
- 1/2 teaspoon nutmeg

Allergens:
- Nuts (almond butter)

DIRECTIONS

1. Preheat the oven to 350°F (175°C) and line a baking sheet with parchment paper.
2. In a large bowl, combine pumpkin puree, oats, honey or maple syrup, melted coconut oil, cinnamon, ginger, and nutmeg. Mix until well combined.
3. Scoop tablespoon-sized balls of dough onto the baking sheet and flatten slightly.
4. Bake for 12-15 minutes until golden brown.
5. Let cool on the baking sheet for 5 minutes before transferring to a wire rack to cool completely.

Buckwheat and Carrot Cake

10 slices | 45 min | Macronutrients (per serving): Calories: 180 | Protein: 4 g Fat: 8 g Carbs: 25 g

INGREDIENTS

- 1 1/2 cups buckwheat flour
- 2 cups grated carrots
- 2 large eggs
- 1/2 cup honey or maple syrup
- 1/4 cup coconut oil, melted
- 1 teaspoon vanilla extract
- 1 teaspoon cinnamon
- 1 teaspoon baking soda
- 1/2 teaspoon ginger
- 1/2 teaspoon nutmeg

Allergens:
- Eggs

DIRECTIONS

1. Preheat the oven to 350°F (175°C) and grease a cake pan.
2. In a large bowl, combine grated carrots, eggs, honey or maple syrup, melted coconut oil, and vanilla extract.
3. In another bowl, mix buckwheat flour, baking soda, cinnamon, ginger, and nutmeg.
4. Add the dry ingredients to the wet ingredients and mix until just combined.
5. Pour the batter into the cake pan. Bake for 30-35 minutes, or until a toothpick comes out clean.
6. Let the cake cool in the pan for 10 minutes before transferring to a wire rack to cool completely.

Baking with Whole Grain Flour

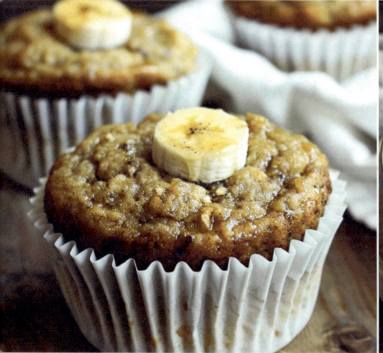

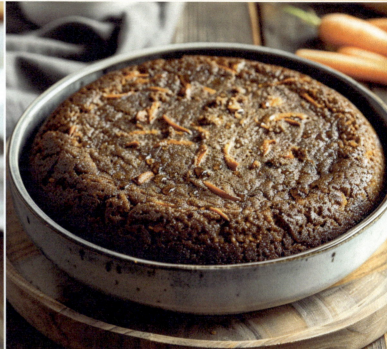

Whole Grain Flour Banana Muffins

12 muffins | 30 min | Macronutrients (per serving): Calories: 180 | Protein: 4 g / Fat: 7 g / Carbs: 25 g

INGREDIENTS

- 2 cups whole grain flour
- 3 ripe bananas, mashed
- 2 large eggs
- 1/4 cup honey or maple syrup
- 1/4 cup coconut oil, melted
- 1 teaspoon vanilla extract
- 1 teaspoon baking soda
- 1/2 teaspoon cinnamon
- 1/4 teaspoon salt

Allergens:
- Eggs

DIRECTIONS

1. Preheat the oven to 350°F (175°C) and line a muffin tin with paper liners.
2. In a large bowl, combine mashed bananas, eggs, honey or maple syrup, melted coconut oil, and vanilla extract.
3. In another bowl, mix whole grain flour, baking soda, cinnamon, and salt.
4. Add the dry ingredients to the wet ingredients and mix until just combined.
5. Fill the muffin cups 3/4 full with batter. Bake for 20-25 minutes, until a toothpick comes out clean.
6. Let muffins cool in the tin for 10 minutes before transferring to a wire rack to cool completely.

Whole Grain Carrot Cake

10 slices | 45 min | Macronutrients (per serving): Calories: 200 | Protein: 5 g / Fat: 8 g / Carbs: 28 g

INGREDIENTS

- 2 cups whole grain flour
- 2 cups grated carrots
- 3 large eggs
- 1/2 cup honey or maple syrup
- 1/4 cup coconut oil, melted
- 1 teaspoon vanilla extract
- 1 teaspoon baking soda
- 1 teaspoon cinnamon
- 1/2 teaspoon nutmeg
- 1/4 teaspoon salt

Allergens:
- Eggs

DIRECTIONS

1. Preheat the oven to 350°F (175°C) and grease a cake pan.
2. In a large bowl, combine grated carrots, eggs, honey or maple syrup, melted coconut oil, and vanilla extract.
3. In another bowl, mix whole grain flour, baking soda, cinnamon, nutmeg, and salt.
4. Add the dry ingredients to the wet and mix until just combined.
5. Pour the batter into the prepared pan. Bake for 30-35 minutes, or until a toothpick comes out clean.
6. Let cool in the pan for 10 minutes before transferring to a wire rack to cool completely.

Baking with Whole Grain Flour

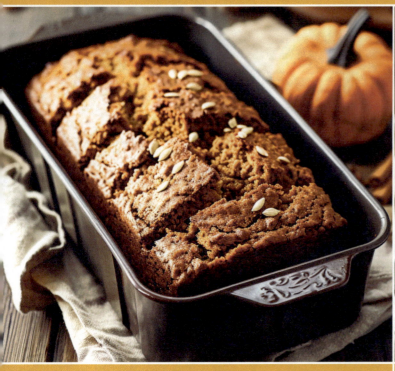

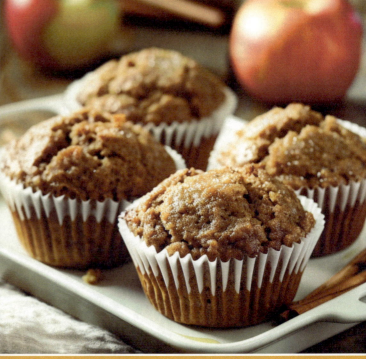

Whole Grain Pumpkin Bread

- 10 slices
- 60 min
- Macronutrients (per serving):
  - Calories: 210
  - Protein: 5 g
  - Fat: 9 g
  - Carbs: 30 g

INGREDIENTS

- 2 cups whole grain flour
- 1 cup pumpkin puree
- 2 large eggs
- 1/4 cup honey or maple syrup
- 1/4 cup coconut oil, melted
- 1 teaspoon vanilla extract
- 1 teaspoon baking soda
- 1 teaspoon cinnamon
- 1/2 teaspoon ginger
- 1/4 teaspoon nutmeg
- 1/4 teaspoon salt

Allergens:
- Eggs

DIRECTIONS

1. Preheat the oven to 350°F (175°C) and grease a loaf pan.
2. In a large bowl, combine pumpkin puree, eggs, honey or maple syrup, melted coconut oil, and vanilla extract.
3. In another bowl, mix whole grain flour, baking soda, cinnamon, ginger, nutmeg, and salt.
4. Add the dry ingredients to the wet ingredients and mix until just combined.
5. Pour the batter into the prepared loaf pan. Bake for 45-50 minutes, or until a toothpick inserted into the center comes out clean.
6. Let the bread cool in the pan for 10 minutes before transferring to a wire rack to cool completely.

Whole Grain Apple Cinnamon Muffins

- 12 muffins
- 30 min
- Macronutrients (per serving):
  - Calories: 170
  - Protein: 4 g
  - Fat: 6 g
  - Carbs: 25 g

INGREDIENTS

- 2 cups whole grain flour
- 1 cup applesauce
- 2 large eggs
- 1/4 cup honey or maple syrup
- 1/4 cup coconut oil, melted
- 1 teaspoon vanilla extract
- 1 teaspoon baking soda
- 1 teaspoon cinnamon
- 1/4 teaspoon salt

Allergens:
- Eggs

DIRECTIONS

1. Preheat the oven to 350°F (175°C) and line a muffin tin with paper liners.
2. In a large bowl, combine applesauce, eggs, honey or maple syrup, melted coconut oil, and vanilla extract.
3. In another bowl, mix whole grain flour, baking soda, cinnamon, and salt.
4. Add the dry ingredients to the wet ingredients and mix until just combined.
5. Fill the muffin cups about 3/4 full with the batter. Bake for 20-25 minutes, or until a toothpick inserted into the center comes out clean.
6. Let the muffins cool in the tin for 10 minutes before transferring to a wire rack to cool completely.

Nut and Seed Desserts

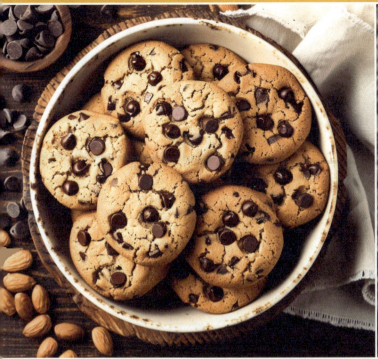

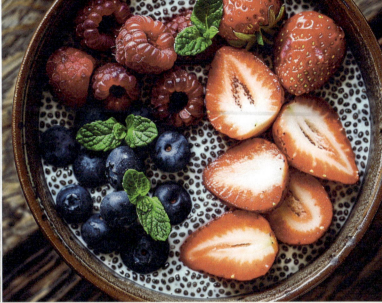

Almond Flour Chocolate Chip Cookies

- 16 cookies
- 20 min
- Macronutrients (per serving):
  - Calories: 150
  - Protein: 3 g
  - Fat: 12 g
  - Carbs: 10 g

INGREDIENTS

- 2 cups almond flour
- 1/4 cup coconut oil, melted
- 1/4 cup honey or maple syrup
- 1 teaspoon vanilla extract
- 1/2 teaspoon baking soda
- 1/4 teaspoon salt
- 1/2 cup dark chocolate chips

Allergens:
- Nuts (almond flour)

DIRECTIONS

1. Preheat the oven to 350°F (175°C) and line a baking sheet with parchment paper.
2. In a large bowl, mix almond flour, coconut oil, honey or maple syrup, vanilla extract, baking soda, and salt until combined.
3. Fold in dark chocolate chips.
4. Scoop tablespoon-sized dough balls onto the baking sheet and flatten slightly.
5. Bake for 10-12 minutes until golden brown at the edges.
6. Cool on the baking sheet for 5 minutes, then transfer to a wire rack to cool completely.

Chia Seed Pudding with Berries

- 4
- 10 min (+ chilling time)
- Macronutrients (per serving):
  - Calories: 200
  - Protein: 5 g
  - Fat: 8 g
  - Carbs: 28 g

INGREDIENTS

- 2 cups plant-based milk (almond, oat, or coconut)
- 1/2 cup chia seeds
- 1/4 cup honey or maple syrup
- 1 teaspoon vanilla extract
- 1 cup mixed berries (blueberries, raspberries, strawberries)

Allergens:
- None (ensure the plant-based milk used is free from allergens you need to avoid)

DIRECTIONS

1. In a bowl, combine plant-based milk, chia seeds, honey or maple syrup, and vanilla extract. Stir well.
2. Cover the bowl and refrigerate for at least 4 hours or overnight until the mixture thickens to a pudding-like consistency.
3. Once the pudding is set, stir in mixed berries.
4. Serve chilled, topping with extra berries if desired.

Nut and Seed Desserts

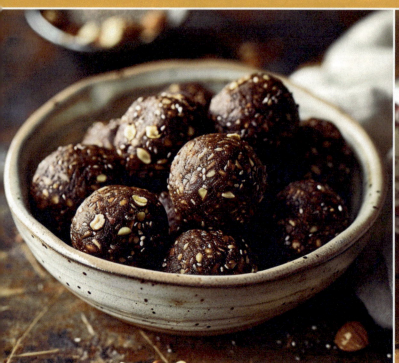

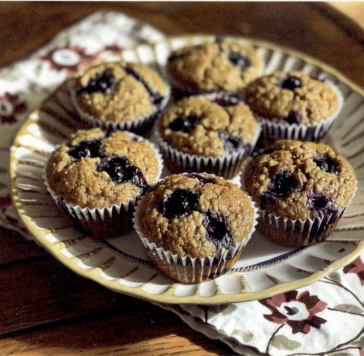

Walnut and Date Energy Balls

20 balls | 10 min (+ chilling time)

Macronutrients (per serving):
Calories: 100
Protein: 2 g
Fat: 7 g
Carbs: 12 g

INGREDIENTS

- 1 cup walnuts
- 1 cup pitted dates
- 1/4 cup chia seeds
- 1/4 cup unsweetened cocoa powder
- 1 tablespoon coconut oil, melted
- 1 teaspoon vanilla extract

Allergens:
- Nuts (walnuts)

DIRECTIONS

1. In a food processor, combine walnuts, dates, chia seeds, cocoa powder, coconut oil, and vanilla extract. Process until the mixture is well combined and sticky.
2. Scoop tablespoon-sized amounts of the mixture and roll into balls.
3. Place the energy balls on a baking sheet and refrigerate for at least 30 minutes to firm up.
4. Store in an airtight container in the refrigerator.

Flaxseed and Blueberry Muffins

12 muffins | 30 min

Macronutrients (per serving):
Calories: 180
Protein: 4 g
Fat: 8 g
Carbs: 24 g

INGREDIENTS

- 2 cups whole grain flour
- 1/4 cup ground flaxseeds
- 1/2 cup honey or maple syrup
- 1/2 cup plant-based milk (almond, oat, or coconut)
- 1/4 cup coconut oil, melted
- 2 large eggs
- 1 teaspoon vanilla extract
- 1 teaspoon baking soda
- 1/2 teaspoon salt
- 1 cup fresh blueberries

Allergens:
- Eggs

DIRECTIONS

1. Preheat the oven to 350°F (175°C) and line a muffin tin with paper liners.
2. In a large bowl, combine honey or maple syrup, plant-based milk, melted coconut oil, eggs, and vanilla extract.
3. In another bowl, mix whole grain flour, ground flaxseeds, baking soda, and salt.
4. Combine dry and wet ingredients, then fold in blueberries.
5. Fill muffin cups 3/4 full and bake for 20-25 minutes until a toothpick comes out clean.
6. Cool in the tin for 10 minutes before transferring to a wire rack to cool completely.

Plant-Based Milk Desserts

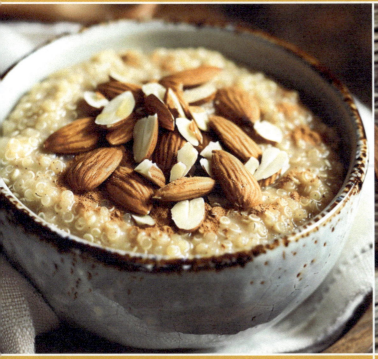
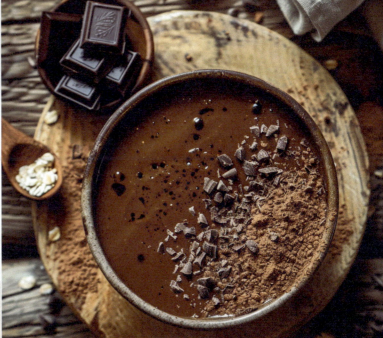

Almond Milk Quinoa Pudding | Oat Milk Chocolate Pudding

Servings: 4 | **Time:** 30 min
Macronutrients (per serving): Calories: 220, Protein: 6 g, Fat: 7 g, Carbs: 35 g

Servings: 4 | **Time:** 10 min (+ chilling time)
Macronutrients (per serving): Calories: 150, Protein: 2 g, Fat: 5 g, Carbs: 28 g

INGREDIENTS (Almond Milk Quinoa Pudding)
- 1 cup quinoa
- 4 cups almond milk
- 1/4 cup honey or maple syrup
- 1 teaspoon vanilla extract
- 1/2 teaspoon cinnamon
- 1/4 teaspoon salt
- 1/4 cup sliced almonds

Allergens:
- Nuts (almond milk, sliced almonds)

INGREDIENTS (Oat Milk Chocolate Pudding)
- 2 cups oat milk
- 1/4 cup cocoa powder
- 1/4 cup honey or maple syrup
- 1/4 cup cornstarch
- 1 teaspoon vanilla extract
- 1/4 teaspoon salt

Allergens:
- None

DIRECTIONS (Almond Milk Quinoa Pudding)
1. Rinse the quinoa under cold water. In a large pot, combine the quinoa and almond milk. Bring to a boil, then reduce heat and simmer for 20-25 minutes until the quinoa is tender and the mixture thickens.
2. Stir in the honey or maple syrup, vanilla extract, cinnamon, and salt. Continue to cook for another 5 minutes until well combined.
3. Serve warm or chilled, topped with sliced almonds.

DIRECTIONS (Oat Milk Chocolate Pudding)
1. In a saucepan, whisk together oat milk, cocoa powder, honey or maple syrup, cornstarch, vanilla extract, and salt until smooth.
2. Place the saucepan over medium heat and cook, stirring constantly, until the mixture comes to a boil and thickens, about 5-7 minutes.
3. Remove from heat and let cool for a few minutes. Transfer to serving bowls and refrigerate for at least 2 hours before serving.
4. Serve chilled.

Plant-Based Milk Desserts

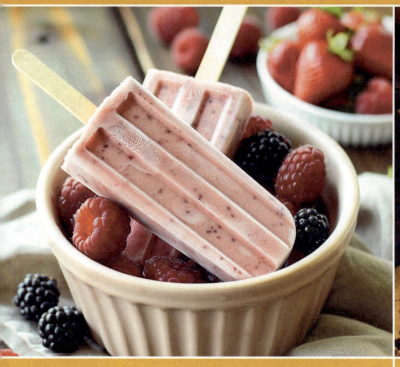

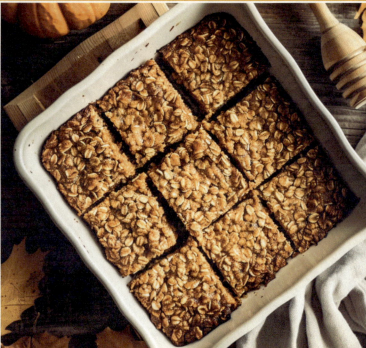

Almond Milk Berry Popsicles

8 popsicles | 10 min (+ chilling time) | Macronutrients (per serving): Calories: 90 | Protein: 1 g Fat: 2 g Carbs: 18 g

INGREDIENTS

- 2 cups almond milk
- 1/2 cup honey or maple syrup
- 1 teaspoon vanilla extract
- 1 cup mixed berries (blueberries, raspberries, strawberries)

Allergens:
- Nuts (almond milk)

DIRECTIONS

1. In a blender, combine almond milk, honey or maple syrup, vanilla extract, and mixed berries. Blend until smooth.
2. Pour the mixture into popsicle molds, leaving a little space at the top for expansion.
3. Insert sticks and freeze for at least 4 hours or until solid.
4. To release the popsicles, run warm water over the outside of the molds for a few seconds.

Pumpkin Spice Oat Bars

16 bars | 40 min | Macronutrients (per serving): Calories: 180 | Protein: 4 g Fat: 7 g Carbs: 30 g

INGREDIENTS

- 1 cup oat milk
- 1/2 cup honey or maple syrup
- 1/4 cup melted coconut oil
- 1 cup pumpkin puree
- 1 tsp vanilla extract
- 2 cups rolled oats
- 1/2 cup whole grain flour
- 1/4 cup chia seeds
- 1 tsp baking powder
- 1 tsp cinnamon
- 1/2 tsp ginger
- 1/2 tsp turmeric
- 1/4 tsp salt

Allergens:
- None

DIRECTIONS

1. Preheat oven to 350°F (175°C) and line a baking dish with parchment paper.
2. In a large bowl, combine oat milk, honey, melted coconut oil, pumpkin puree, and vanilla extract.
3. In another bowl, mix rolled oats, whole grain flour, chia seeds, baking powder, cinnamon, ginger, turmeric, and salt.
4. Add dry ingredients to wet and mix well. Pour into the baking dish and spread evenly.
5. Bake for 25-30 minutes, until edges are golden and a toothpick comes out clean. Cool completely before cutting into squares.

FESTIVE DISHES TAILORED FOR AN ANTI-INFLAMMATORY DIET

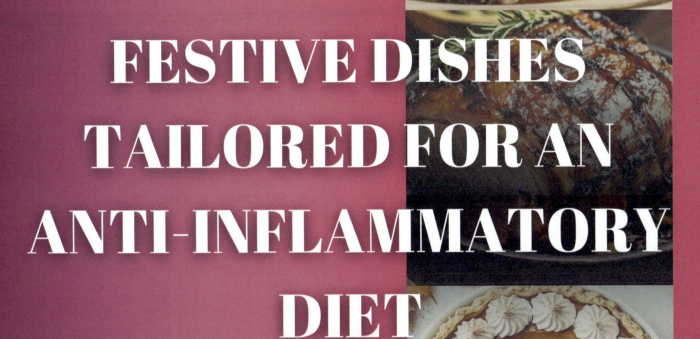

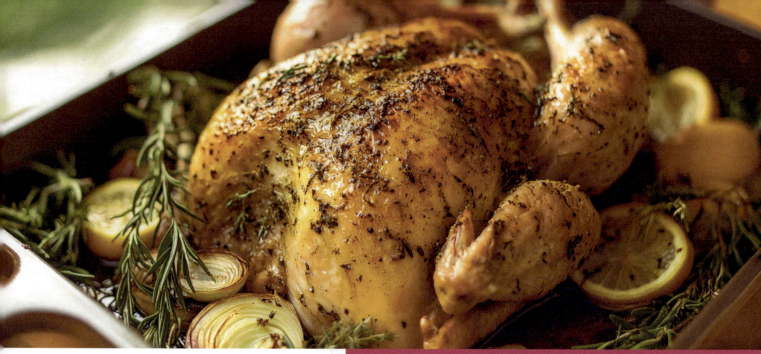

| 8 | 3.5 hrs | Macronutrients (per serving): Calories: 320 | Protein: 40 g Fat: 16 g Carbs: 2 g |

Anti-Inflammatory Roast Turkey

INGREDIENTS

- 1 whole turkey (10-12 pounds), preferably organic and free-range
- 2 tablespoons olive oil
- 1 teaspoon turmeric
- 1 teaspoon ground ginger
- 1 teaspoon garlic powder
- 1 teaspoon onion powder
- 1 teaspoon rosemary (fresh or dried)
- 1 teaspoon thyme (fresh or dried)
- 1 teaspoon sea salt
- 1/2 teaspoon black pepper
- 1 lemon, halved
- 1 onion, quartered
- 3-4 garlic cloves, whole
- 2 cups low-sodium chicken broth (or water)

DIRECTIONS

1. Preheat your oven to 325°F (165°C).
2. Remove the giblets and neck, rinse with cold water, and pat dry. Place the turkey on a roasting rack in a large pan.
3. Mix olive oil, turmeric, ground ginger, garlic powder, onion powder, rosemary, thyme, salt, and pepper. Rub the mixture all over the turkey, including under the skin. Place lemon halves, onion quarters, and garlic cloves inside the cavity.
4. Pour chicken broth into the pan for moisture, cover the turkey with foil, and roast for 2.5 to 3 hours at 165°F (74°C). Remove foil for the last 30 minutes to brown the skin.
5. Once done, remove the turkey from the oven and let it rest for 20 minutes before carving. Resting helps the juices redistribute throughout the meat, making it more tender.
6. Carve the turkey and serve with your favorite anti-inflammatory sides, such as roasted vegetables or a quinoa salad.

HELPFUL TIPS

- *Brining the Turkey:* If you have time, brine the turkey overnight in a solution of water, salt, and herbs to enhance flavor and moisture.
- *Use of Herbs:* Fresh herbs add more flavor and anti-inflammatory benefits, so use them if available.
- *Avoid Processed Ingredients:* Stick to natural, whole foods to maintain the anti-inflammatory benefits of this recipe.

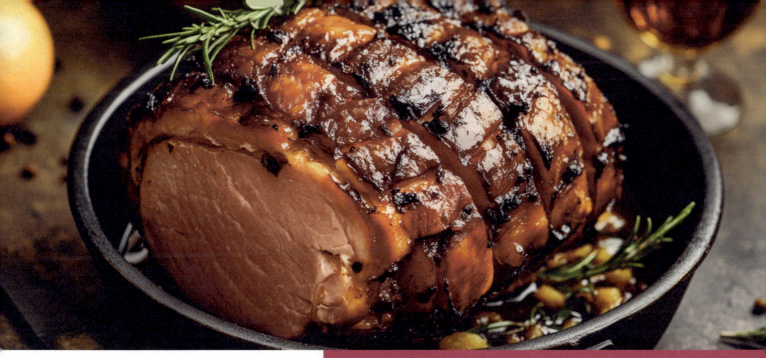

8 | **2 hrs 15 min** | Macronutrients (per serving): Calories: 320 | Protein: 25 g Fat: 18 g Carbs: 12 g

Anti-Inflammatory Baked Ham

INGREDIENTS

- 4 lbs uncured, nitrate-free ham
- 1/4 cup pure maple syrup
- 2 tbsp Dijon mustard
- 1 tbsp apple cider vinegar
- 1/2 tsp ground ginger
- 1/2 tsp ground cinnamon
- 1/4 tsp ground cloves
- 1 tbsp olive oil
- 1/2 cup fresh orange juice
- 2 tsp fresh rosemary, finely chopped

DIRECTIONS

1. Preheat your oven to 325°F (163°C).
2. Place the ham in a roasting pan, fat side up. If your ham has a thick layer of fat, you can score it with a knife to allow the glaze to penetrate.
3. In a small bowl, whisk together the maple syrup, Dijon mustard, apple cider vinegar, ground ginger, ground cinnamon, ground cloves, and olive oil until well combined.
4. Brush the glaze generously over the ham, making sure to cover all sides.
5. Pour the fresh orange juice into the bottom of the roasting pan to keep the ham moist while roasting. Cover the ham loosely with foil.
6. Roast the ham in the preheated oven for about 1.5 to 2 hours (about 20 minutes per pound), basting with the pan juices every 30 minutes.
7. During the last 30 minutes of cooking, remove the foil to allow the ham to caramelize and develop a rich, golden-brown crust.
8. Remove the ham from the oven and let it rest for 10-15 minutes before slicing. Garnish with freshly chopped rosemary.

HELPFUL TIPS

- *Choose Quality Ham:* Choose an uncured, nitrate-free ham to avoid harmful preservatives.
- *Monitor the Temperature:* A meat thermometer ensures the ham reaches 140°F (60°C) internally.
- *Pairing:* Pair with anti-inflammatory sides like roasted Brussels sprouts, sweet potatoes, or a fresh green salad with lemon vinaigrette.

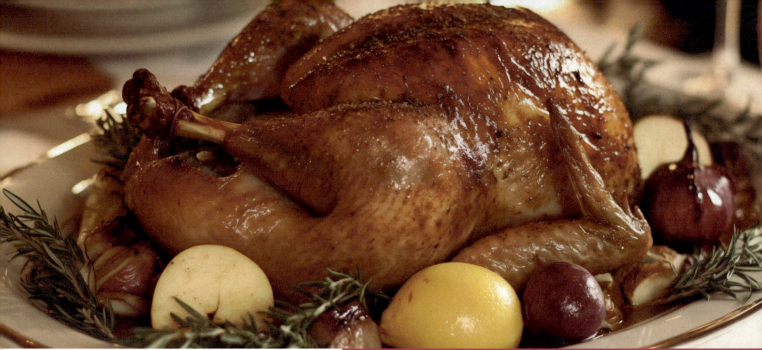

		Macronutrients (per serving):	Protein: 25 g
6	2 hrs 15 min	Calories: 350	Fat: 25 g Carbs: 8 g

Roast Duck (or Goose) for Thanksgiving

INGREDIENTS

- 1 whole duck or goose (about 4-5 lbs)
- 1 tablespoon olive oil (extra virgin)
- 2 teaspoons turmeric powder
- 1 teaspoon ground ginger
- 1 teaspoon dried rosemary
- 1 teaspoon thyme
- 1/2 teaspoon black pepper
- 1/2 teaspoon sea salt
- 2 lemons, quartered
- 2 apples, quartered
- 4 garlic cloves, smashed
- 1 small onion, quartered
- Fresh herbs for garnish (optional: parsley, thyme, or rosemary)
- 1 cup water or low-sodium chicken broth

DIRECTIONS

1. Preheat to 350°F (175°C).
2. Prepare the Duck/Goose: Rinse, pat dry, and trim excess fat. Rub with seasoning (olive oil, turmeric, ginger, rosemary, thyme, pepper, salt). Stuff the cavity with lemon, apple, garlic, and onion.
3. Roast: Place on a rack in a roasting pan. Add water or broth to the pan. Roast for 2-2.5 hours, basting every 30 minutes, until internal temperature reaches 165°F (74°C).
4. Optional Crispy Skin: Increase temperature to 400°F (200°C) for the last 10-15 minutes for extra crispiness.
5. Rest and Serve: Let rest for 15 minutes, then carve. Garnish with fresh herbs and serve.

HELPFUL TIPS

- *Spices:* Turmeric and ginger provide anti-inflammatory benefits.
- *Healthy Fats:* Olive oil promotes heart health.
- *Moisture:* Baste regularly to keep the meat tender.

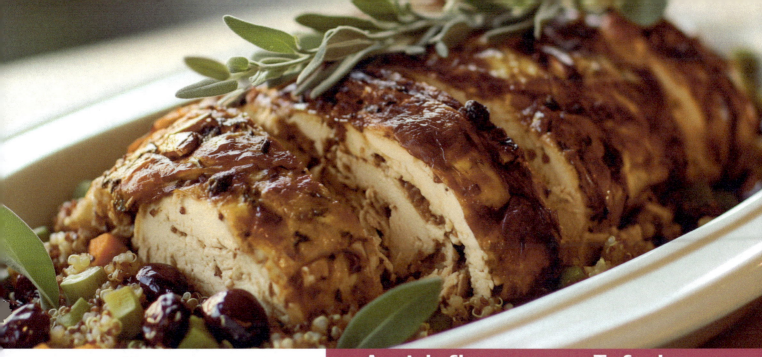

Anti-Inflammatory Tofurkey (Tofu Turkey)

Servings: 6 | **Time:** 2 hrs 15 min | **Macronutrients (per serving):** Calories: 220, Protein: 15 g, Fat: 14 g, Carbs: 12 g

INGREDIENTS

- 2 blocks (16 oz each) firm organic tofu
- 1 tablespoon olive oil (extra virgin)
- 1/4 cup ground flaxseeds
- 1/2 cup vegetable broth (low-sodium)
- 1 tablespoon tamari (or coconut aminos)
- 1 teaspoon turmeric powder
- 1 teaspoon garlic powder
- 1 teaspoon onion powder
- 1 teaspoon dried thyme
- 1 teaspoon dried rosemary
- 1 teaspoon ground ginger
- 1 tablespoon lemon juice
- 1/4 cup ground walnuts (optional)

For the Stuffing:

- 1/2 cup cooked quinoa or wild rice
- 1/2 cup diced celery, carrots, and onions
- 1 tablespoon olive oil
- 1/4 cup chopped dried cranberries (optional)
- 1 teaspoon dried sage
- 1/2 teaspoon black pepper and sea salt

DIRECTIONS

1. Prepare the Tofu: Drain and press tofu for 20 minutes. Blend with flaxseeds, tamari, spices, and lemon juice until smooth.
2. Prepare the Stuffing: Sauté onions, carrots, and celery in olive oil. Add quinoa or rice, cranberries, sage, salt, and pepper. Cook for 2-3 minutes.
3. Assemble the Tofurkey: Line a bowl with plastic wrap. Spread two-thirds of the tofu mixture along the sides. Fill with stuffing, cover with remaining tofu, and refrigerate for 1 hour.
4. Bake: Preheat oven to 375°F (190°C). Invert the tofu onto a baking sheet, brush with olive oil, and bake for 45-50 minutes.
5. Serve: Let the tofurkey cool for 10 minutes before slicing. Serve with anti-inflammatory sides like roasted sweet potatoes or steamed broccoli.

HELPFUL TIPS

- For a chewier texture, freeze tofu overnight before pressing.
- Customize the stuffing with ingredients like spinach or walnuts.
- Leftovers can be stored in the fridge for up to 3 days.

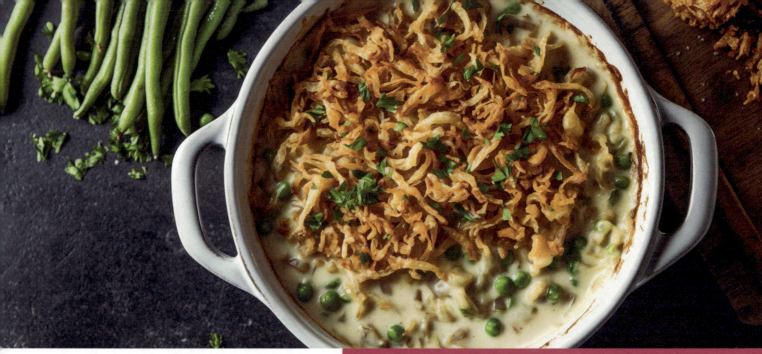

| 🍴 6 | 🕐 45 min | Macronutrients (per serving): Calories: 180 | Protein: 4 g Fat: 8 g Carbs: 22 g |

Green Bean Casserole with Crispy Onions and Creamy Soup

INGREDIENTS

- 1 lb (450g) fresh green beans, trimmed and cut into 2-inch pieces
- 1 cup (240ml) unsweetened almond milk or oat milk
- 1 cup (240ml) low-sodium vegetable broth
- 1/4 cup (30g) whole wheat flour or almond flour (for gluten-free option)
- 1 small yellow onion, finely chopped
- 2 cloves garlic, minced
- 1 tbsp extra virgin olive oil
- 1/4 tsp ground turmeric
- 1/4 tsp ground black pepper
- 1/4 tsp sea salt (optional)
- 1/2 cup (50g) crispy fried onions (preferably homemade or gluten-free)
- 1/4 cup (30g) chopped fresh parsley (optional, for garnish)
- 1 tbsp nutritional yeast (optional, for a cheesy flavor)

HELPFUL TIPS

- *Avoid Soggy Onions: To keep the crispy onions on top from getting soggy, wait until the last 5-10 minutes of baking to add them. This will ensure they stay crunchy and golden.*

DIRECTIONS

1. Preheat your oven to 375°F (190°C).
2. Bring a large pot of water to a boil. Add the green beans and blanch for 3-4 minutes until they are tender-crisp. Drain and immediately transfer to a bowl of ice water to stop the cooking process. Drain again and set aside.
3. Prepare the Creamy Soup Base: In a medium saucepan, heat the olive oil over medium heat. Add the chopped onion and garlic, sauté until softened, about 3-4 minutes. Stir in the flour and cook for 1 minute to eliminate the raw taste. Gradually whisk in the almond milk and vegetable broth, stirring constantly to avoid lumps. Cook for 5-7 minutes until the mixture thickens into a creamy consistency. Stir in the turmeric, black pepper, and sea salt (if using).
4. Assemble the Casserole: In a large mixing bowl, combine the blanched green beans with the creamy soup mixture. Stir until the beans are evenly coated. Transfer the mixture to a lightly greased 9x9-inch (23x23 cm) baking dish. Sprinkle the crispy fried onions evenly over the top.
5. Bake the Casserole: Bake in the preheated oven for 20-25 minutes until the casserole is bubbly and the onions are golden brown.
6. Serve: Let the casserole cool for a few minutes before serving. Garnish with chopped fresh parsley and a sprinkle of nutritional yeast, if desired.

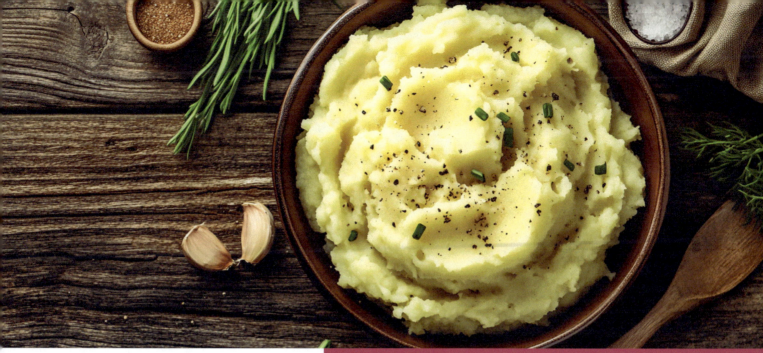

Anti-Inflammatory Mashed Potatoes

 4 | 30 min | Macronutrients (per serving): Calories: 150 | Protein: 3 g Fat: 4 g Carbs: 28 g

INGREDIENTS

- 4 medium russet or Yukon Gold potatoes, peeled and chopped
- 1/2 cup unsweetened almond milk (or any other plant-based milk)
- 2 tablespoons extra-virgin olive oil
- 1 tablespoon nutritional yeast (optional, for a cheesy flavor)
- 1/2 teaspoon garlic powder
- 1/2 teaspoon onion powder
- Sea salt and black pepper to taste
- Fresh chives or parsley for garnish (optional)

DIRECTIONS

1. Cook the Potatoes: Place the chopped potatoes in a large pot and cover with cold water. Add a pinch of sea salt to the water. Bring the water to a boil over medium-high heat. Reduce the heat and simmer until the potatoes are tender when pierced with a fork, about 15-20 minutes. Drain the potatoes and return them to the pot.
2. Mash the Potatoes: Using a potato masher or a hand mixer, mash the potatoes until smooth. Slowly add the almond milk and olive oil, continuing to mash until the potatoes reach your desired consistency.
3. Season the Potatoes: Stir in the garlic powder, onion powder, nutritional yeast (if using), sea salt, and black pepper. Adjust the seasoning to taste.
4. Serve: Transfer the mashed potatoes to a serving bowl. If desired, garnish with fresh chives or parsley. Serve hot, with an extra drizzle of olive oil on top if desired.

HELPFUL TIPS

- *Choosing Potatoes:* Yukon Gold potatoes are great for this recipe because of their naturally creamy texture, which helps achieve that perfect mashed potato consistency.
- *Nutritional Yeast:* This ingredient adds a cheesy flavor without dairy, making it a great option for those following an anti-inflammatory diet.
- *Serving Suggestions:* Serve these mashed potatoes as a side dish to roasted vegetables or lean protein like grilled chicken or turkey breast.

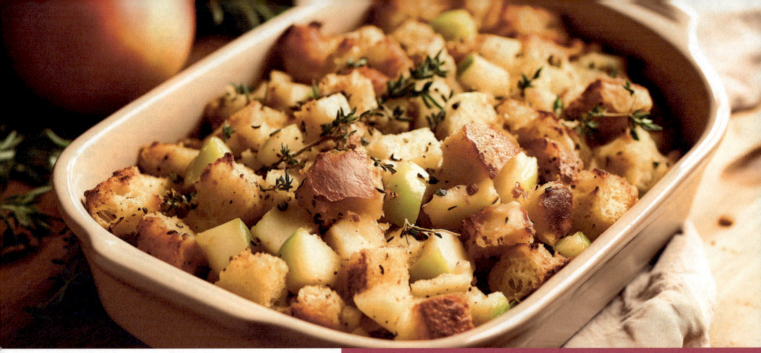

Anti-Inflammatory Stuffing (Dressing)

 6 | 60-75 min | **Macronutrients (per serving):** Calories: 180 | Protein: 4 g Fat: 6 g Carbs: 28 g

INGREDIENTS

- 6 cups cubed whole-grain or gluten-free bread (preferably sprouted or sourdough)
- 2 tablespoons extra-virgin olive oil
- 1 medium onion, finely chopped
- 3 stalks celery, chopped
- 3 cloves garlic, minced
- 1 large apple, peeled and diced
- 1/4 cup fresh parsley, chopped
- 1 tablespoon fresh rosemary, chopped
- 1 tablespoon fresh thyme, chopped
- 1 teaspoon dried sage
- 1/4 teaspoon turmeric (for added anti-inflammatory benefits)
- 1/4 teaspoon black pepper
- 1/2 teaspoon sea salt
- 1 1/2 cups low-sodium vegetable broth
- 1/4 cup walnuts or pecans (optional, for crunch and extra omega-3s)

HELPFUL TIPS

- *Make it Ahead:* You can prepare this stuffing a day in advance and reheat it in the oven before serving.
- *Customizable:* Feel free to add other anti-inflammatory ingredients like chopped kale or dried cranberries for extra flavor and texture.

DIRECTIONS

1. Prepare the Bread. Preheat your oven to 350°F (175°C). Spread the cubed bread on a baking sheet and toast in the oven for about 10-15 minutes, or until slightly crispy. Set aside to cool.
2. Sauté the Vegetables. In a large skillet, heat the olive oil over medium heat. Add the chopped onion, celery, and garlic, and sauté for about 5-7 minutes, or until softened and fragrant. Add the diced apple and continue cooking for another 2-3 minutes.
3. In a large mixing bowl, combine the toasted bread cubes with the sautéed vegetables and apple. Add the fresh parsley, rosemary, thyme, sage, turmeric, black pepper, and sea salt. Stir to combine. Gradually pour in the vegetable broth while stirring until the bread is moistened but not soggy.
4. If using, fold in the chopped walnuts or pecans for added texture and healthy fats.
5. Transfer the stuffing mixture to a lightly greased baking dish (if you're not stuffing it into a turkey). Cover with foil and bake in the preheated oven for 25 minutes.
6. Remove the foil and bake for an additional 10-15 minutes, or until the top is golden and crispy.
7. Let the stuffing cool slightly before serving. It can be enjoyed as a side dish with turkey or on its own.

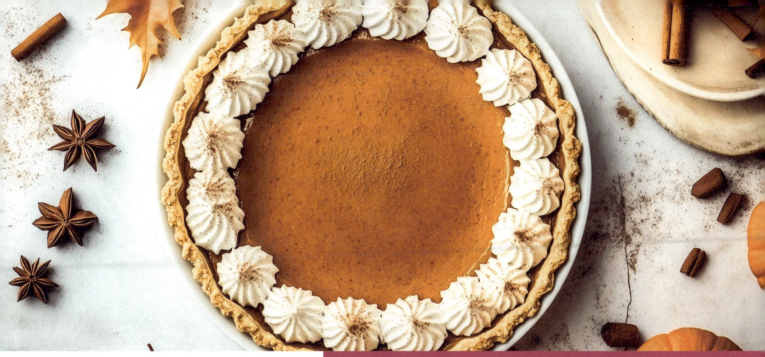

Anti-Inflammatory Pumpkin Pie

Serves: 8 | **Time:** 1 hr 45 min
Macronutrients (per serving): Calories: 210 | Protein: 5 g | Fat: 10 g | Carbs: 28 g

INGREDIENTS

For the Crust:
- 1 cup almond flour
- 1/4 cup coconut flour
- 1/4 cup coconut oil, melted
- 1 tablespoon maple syrup
- 1/2 teaspoon cinnamon
- 1/4 teaspoon sea salt

For the Filling:
- 1 1/2 cups pumpkin puree (canned or homemade)
- 1/2 cup coconut milk (full-fat)
- 2 large eggs
- 1/4 cup maple syrup
- 1 teaspoon vanilla extract
- 1 teaspoon ground cinnamon
- 1/2 teaspoon ground ginger
- 1/4 teaspoon ground nutmeg
- 1/4 teaspoon ground cloves
- 1/8 teaspoon ground turmeric (optional, for added anti-inflammatory benefit)
- 1/8 teaspoon black pepper (enhances absorption of turmeric)

DIRECTIONS

1. Prepare the Crust:
- Preheat the oven to 350°F (175°C).
- Mix almond flour, coconut flour, melted coconut oil, maple syrup, cinnamon, and sea salt in a bowl until a dough forms.
- Press the dough into a 9-inch pie dish.
- Bake for 10 minutes, then set aside.

2. Make the Filling:
- Whisk together the pumpkin puree, coconut milk, eggs, maple syrup, vanilla, and spices until smooth.
- Pour the filling into the crust and smooth the top.

3. Bake the Pie:
- Bake for 45-50 minutes, or until the filling is set and a toothpick comes out clean.
- Let the pie cool completely before slicing.

4. Serve with coconut whipped cream if desired.

HELPFUL TIPS

- *Coconut Milk: Adds creaminess to the filling without dairy, making it easier on digestion and supporting an anti-inflammatory diet.*
- *Turmeric & Black Pepper: Turmeric is known for its anti-inflammatory properties, and black pepper enhances its absorption. These spices add a subtle flavor that complements the traditional pumpkin pie spices.*

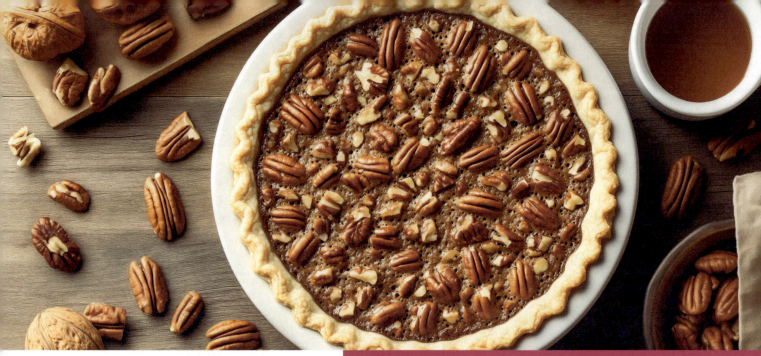

Anti-Inflammatory Pecan Pie

 8 | ⏱ 2 hrs | Macronutrients (per serving): Calories: 320 | Protein: 5 g Fat: 22 g Carbs: 28 g

INGREDIENTS

For the Crust:
- 1 1/2 cups almond flour
- 1/4 cup coconut flour
- 1/4 cup melted coconut oil
- 2 tbsp maple syrup (pure)
- 1/4 tsp sea salt

For the Filling:
- 1 1/2 cups raw pecans
- 3/4 cup pure maple syrup
- 1/4 cup coconut sugar
- 1/4 cup unsweetened almond milk
- 1/4 cup melted coconut oil
- 2 large eggs
- 1 tsp vanilla extract
- 1/2 tsp ground cinnamon
- 1/4 tsp sea salt

HELPFUL TIPS

- *For a richer flavor:* Toast the pecans lightly before adding them to the filling. This enhances the nutty flavor.
- *Substitute sweeteners:* If you prefer, you can substitute the maple syrup with honey, but be mindful of the different glycemic impacts.

DIRECTIONS

1. Prepare the Crust:
- Preheat your oven to 350°F (175°C).
- In a mixing bowl, combine the almond flour, coconut flour, melted coconut oil, maple syrup, and sea salt. Mix until well combined and a dough forms.
- Press the dough evenly into the bottom and up the sides of a 9-inch pie dish. Use a fork to prick the bottom of the crust a few times to prevent bubbling.
- Bake the crust for about 10-12 minutes until lightly golden. Remove from the oven and let it cool.

2. Prepare the Filling:
- In a large bowl, whisk together the maple syrup, coconut sugar, almond milk, melted coconut oil, eggs, vanilla extract, cinnamon, and sea salt until well combined.
- Stir in the pecans, ensuring they are well coated with the mixture.

3. Assemble and Bake:
- Pour the pecan filling into the cooled crust.
- Bake the pie at 350°F (175°C) for 40-45 minutes, or until the filling is set and the top is golden.
- If the crust edges start to brown too quickly, cover them with foil.

4. Cool and Serve:
- Allow the pie to cool completely before serving. This will help the filling set properly.

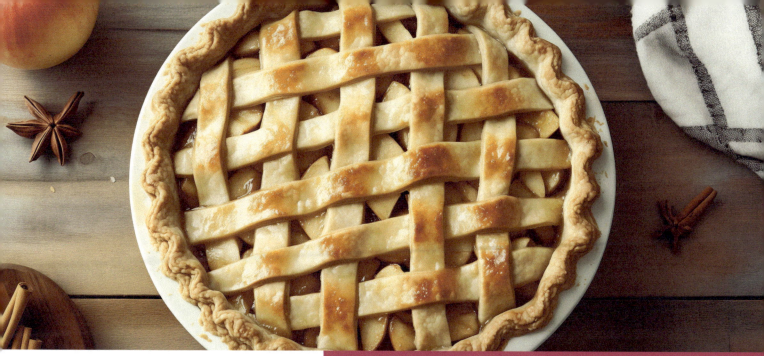

Anti-Inflammatory Apple Pie

Serves: 8 | Time: 2 hrs 20 min
Macronutrients (per serving): Calories: 220 | Protein: 3 g | Fat: 8 g | Carbs: 35 g

INGREDIENTS

For the Crust:
- 1 1/2 cups almond flour
- 1/2 cup oat flour (gluten-free if needed)
- 1/4 cup cold coconut oil, solid
- 2 tbsp pure maple syrup
- 1/4 tsp sea salt
- 3-4 tbsp cold water

For the Filling:
- 5 medium apples (Granny Smith or Honeycrisp), peeled, cored, and thinly sliced
- 1/4 cup pure maple syrup
- 1 tbsp lemon juice
- 2 tbsp arrowroot powder or cornstarch
- 1 1/2 tsp ground cinnamon
- 1/4 tsp ground ginger
- 1/4 tsp ground nutmeg
- 1/4 tsp ground turmeric (optional, for added anti-inflammatory benefits)
- 1/2 tsp vanilla extract

DIRECTIONS

1. Prepare the Crust:
   - Combine almond flour, oat flour, and sea salt in a bowl.
   - Add cold coconut oil and mix until the mixture resembles coarse crumbs.
   - Add maple syrup and cold water gradually until the dough holds together.
   - Divide into two portions, wrap, and refrigerate for 30 minutes.
2. Prepare the Filling:
   - Toss apple slices with lemon juice, then add maple syrup, arrowroot, spices, and vanilla extract. Set aside.
3. Assemble the Pie:
   - Preheat oven to 375°F (190°C).
   - Roll out one dough portion and press into a 9-inch pie dish.
   - Add the apple filling, then top with the second rolled-out dough. Seal and cut slits for steam.
4. Bake for 45-50 minutes until the crust is golden and filling is bubbling. Cover edges with foil if they brown too quickly.
5. Let cool for 30 minutes before slicing.

HELPFUL TIPS

- Apples: Use Granny Smith for tartness or Honeycrisp for sweetness.
- Crust: Adjust the top crust as desired (lattice or full cover).

A NOTE OF THANKS

Congratulations on completing the Anti-Inflammatory Diet Cookbook! You've taken a significant step toward improving your health and well-being through mindful eating and nutritious choices. By embracing an anti-inflammatory diet, you've nourished your body with wholesome foods and laid the foundation for a healthier, happier life.

Your journey to better health celebrates the positive changes you've made. Each meal prepared, each new recipe tried, and each day of mindfully eating is a testament to your commitment to wellness. Remember, this journey is not about perfection but progress. Celebrate the small victories and the improvements in your health, energy levels, and overall well-being.

This cookbook has provided you with various delicious recipes and practical tips to make healthy eating enjoyable and sustainable. As you continue to explore and experiment with different foods, remember that flexibility and adaptability are key. Listen to your body, adjust the meal plans to suit your needs, and don't be afraid to try new things. Lastly, recognize that the benefits of an anti-inflammatory diet extend beyond the physical. A balanced diet can enhance your mood, boost your energy, and contribute to a more positive outlook

on life. By nurturing your body with the right foods, you also nurture your mind and spirit.

Celebrate your achievements, no matter how small they may seem, and continue to build on the healthy habits you've developed. Your journey to better health is ongoing, and every step you take is a step towards a vibrant, energized, and fulfilling life!

Your feedback is incredibly important to us. If you enjoyed the book and found it helpful, please consider leaving a review. Your thoughts and experiences help others discover the benefits of an anti-inflammatory diet and motivate us to continue creating useful content.

Made in the USA
Columbia, SC
22 March 2025